AF342044

Fluid Sterilization by Filtration

Third Edition

Fluid Sterilization by Filtration

Third Edition

Peter R. Johnston

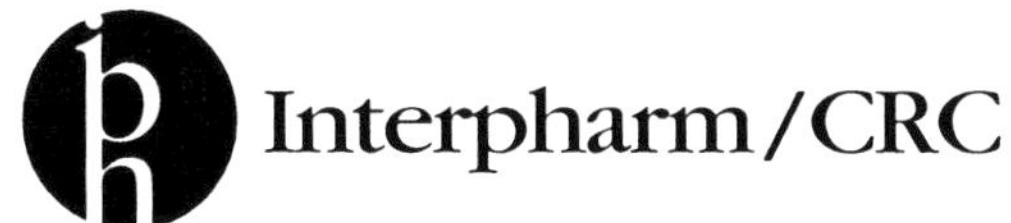

Interpharm/CRC

Boca Raton   London   New York   Washington, D.C.

First Indian Reprint, 2016

Library of Congress Cataloging-in-Publication Data

Johnston, Peter R.
    Fluid sterilization by filtration / Peter R. Johnston. -- 3rd ed.
      p. cm.
    Previous editions have subtitle: the filter integrity test and other filtration topics.
    Includes bibliographical references and index.
    ISBN 0-8493-1977-3 (alk. paper)
    1. Drugs--Sterilization. 2. Filters and filtration. 3. Sterilization. I. Title.

RS199.S73J64 2003
615′.19--dc22   2003055737

This book contains information obtained from authentic and highly regarded sources. Reprinted material is quoted with permission, and sources are indicated. A wide variety of references are listed. Reasonable efforts have been made to publish reliable data and information, but the author and the publisher cannot assume responsibility for the validity of all materials or for the consequences of their use.

Neither this book nor any part may be reproduced or transmitted in any form or by any means, electronic or mechanical, including photocopying, microfilming, and recording, or by any information storage or retrieval system, without prior permission in writing from the publisher.

The consent of CRC Press LLC does not extend to copying for general distribution, for promotion, for creating new works, or for resale. Specific permission must be obtained in writing from CRC Press LLC for such copying.

Direct all inquiries to CRC Press LLC, 2000 N.W. Corporate Blvd., Boca Raton, Florida 33431.

Trademark Notice: Product or corporate names may be trademarks or registered trademarks, and are used only for identification and explanation, without intent to infringe.

Visit the CRC Press Web site at www.crcpress.com

© 2004 by CRC Press LLC

International Standard Book Number 0-8493-1977-3
Library of Congress Card Number 2003055737
Printed and bound in India by Bhavish Graphics.

For sale in India, Pakistan, Nepal, Bhutan, Bangladesh and Sri Lanka only.

Preface

The first edition of this book, published in 1992 by Interpharm Press with a different subtitle, evolved from talks I made before a 1991 meeting of the Parenteral Drug Association. Theodore Meltzer, chair of that meeting, and editor of the massive *Filtration in the Pharmaceutical Industry*, published by Marcel Dekker in 1986, graciously introduced me to Interpharm.

From 1977 to 1992, I chaired an American Society for Testing and Materials (ASTM) subcommittee on liquid filtration. We wrote about 15 filtration test methods. During 1986, ASTM sponsored a symposium on filtration and published the proceedings in *Special Technical Publication (STP) 975*, in two volumes, one on gas filtration, the other on liquid filtration. Ted Meltzer then introduced me to Tall Oaks Publishing, who, in 1990, brought out my *Fundamentals of Fluid Filtration, a Technical Primer*.

In 1992, the American Filtration and Separation Society (AFS), looking beyond ASTM methods, put out a call for test methods. I collected those methods and other methods and wrote *A Survey of Test Methods in Fluid Filtration*, which was published in 1995 by Gulf Publishing Co. After that press run sold out, Gulf declined to publish an updated second edition. With Gulf's permission, I used information in *Survey* to write a 1998 second edition of *Fundamentals*, which was published in 1998.

In 2001 Mark Jornitz and Ted Meltzer wrote *Sterile Filtration: A Practical Approach*, published by Marcel Dekker. While that work does indeed cover information newer than Meltzer's 1987 book, there are matters that are not included in it that I believe are important for a thorough understanding of the subject. Meanwhile, CRC Press had acquired Interpharm. CRC agreed to publish the present book, the third edition of my *Fluid Sterilization by Filtration*.

The Author

Peter R. Johnston, P.E. was trained in chemistry. After a 1952 Army combat tour in Korea as a platoon leader, he began doing R&D work in the chemical process industry and obtained patents in three different fields of chemistry.

In 1972 his work led him into the filtration business. He became a charter member of ASTM's Committee 21 on Filtration, and for 15 years he chaired the subcommittee on liquid filtration, guiding that group into writing about 15 test methods. ASTM elected him a Fellow.

Johnston has published more than three dozen papers on filtration in a variety of journals and has spoken at many technical meetings. He retired from industry in 1992 and now consults with a variety of people on questions about filtration. He continues to write papers on the subject and reviews papers for publication.

Introduction

A membrane filter medium, meant to sterilize a clear or nearly particle free pharmaceutical liquid, is employed in the final filtration step, just before the operation of filling vials or bottles. But, before that final filtration step, the liquid has already undergone previous filtration with ordinary fibrous filter media. Such previous steps reduce any debris that would quickly clog a membrane filter. Thus, while this book aims at the final filtration step it also addresses the general subject of filtration. Indeed, in some cases that will be discussed, the product to be recovered from a liquid suspension is a powder.

Materials of Construction

When selecting a filter medium, the first thing to consider is the material of construction. The medium must stand up to the fluid to be filtered. Suppliers of membrane filters provide lists of fluids that can be used with each of their products and point out fluids that must not be used with some. Furthermore, suppliers will gladly test any special fluid for compatibility.

The Integrity Test

In the pharmaceutical industry, regulations require that a membrane filter medium meant to sterilize a stream be tested for integrity before and after filtration, to make sure no fluid will or has leaked around it. The integrity test is sometimes called the diffusive flow test, the forward-flow test, the pressure hold test, or the flow decay test. It is performed with the bubble-point test. Instruments are commercially available to perform such tests, along with directions for performing them. By following these procedures and recording the results, operators fulfill the requirements of good manufacturing procedures.

Yet beyond merely following procedures, the alert operator will understand what the procedures and instruments actually measure and do not measure and what the results actually mean. Furthermore, to avoid being misled, the alert investigator will understand the method by which any instrument he or she uses derives results from measurements.

Pore Size

The results of bubble-point tests point to the size of the largest pores. Yet, there is ambiguity in this method, which has yet to be standardized. One investigator's largest pore differs from another's. Similarly, one investigator's absolute filtration differs from another's.

Since the largest pores carry only a very small fraction of the stream, a more important measure of pore size is the flow-averaged diameter, defined by a fluid during flow through the medium. The largest pores on the surface do not extend into the depth of the medium. Yet, when the bubble-point test is correctly performed, it does give an indication of the diameter of the flow-averaged pore. That is, in the random array of pore sizes, the largest pore on the surface is about three times the diameter of the flow-averaged pore.

The flow-averaged pore size is larger than the volume-averaged pore size, which is larger than the number-averaged pore size. Yet, filtration efficiency, while related to pore size, is also related to the thickness of the filter and to the internal surface area, among many other variables.

Rated Pore Size

Aside from pore size, distribution of pore sizes, and the thickness of the filter membrane, the drug manufacturer simply wants a membrane to stop a certain sized microbe. Hence, membranes are rated by a somewhat standardized test that determines if a specific test microbe is stopped with great efficiency. When it does, the membrane is rated for that microbe. Thus, writers employ correct terminology when they speak of, say, a 0.45-μm rated membrane. The rating does not mean the membrane has a pore diameter, whatever that means, of 0.45 μm.

The 0.45-μm rating indicates a membrane stops *Serratia marcescens* with great efficiency. That is, when feeding 10^7 microbes per square centimeter of membrane surface, less than one such microbe appears in the filtrate. Such membranes were once used for sterilizing filtration, but it was found that some filtrates were not sterile. The microbe passing was cultured as *Pseudomonas diminuta* and then used to rate membranes as 0.20 μm (or 0.22 μm, as if the difference is significant). This rating was apparently assigned to show that such a membrane has half the rating of 0.45 μm, even though *Pseudomonas diminuta* (now called *Brevundimonas diminuta*), so cultured, is actually $^4/_5$ the diameter of *Serratia marcescens*. The viscous flow-averaged pore diameter of a 0.45-μm-rated membrane is near 0.85 μm. The viscous flow-averaged pore diameter of a 0.20-μm-rated membrane is near 0.55 μm.

Compared to suppliers of paper and other nonwoven fibrous filter media, suppliers of membrane filters are straightforward in reporting fundamental facts about their membranes. They report thickness, porosity (ratio of void volume to bulk volume), and the flow rate of water under a given driving pressure. From such data, we can deduce the permeability and, thus, the flow-averaged pore diameter. Since most membrane filters are of equal thickness, filtration efficiency is then a simple function of the flow-averaged pore diameter. But filtration efficiency varies with changing membrane materials, as well as with changing fluid-flow rate, viscosity, temperature, and properties of the microbes and particles to be separated.

Someday, perhaps, suppliers of fibrous filter media will report such fundamental data. They generally do report thickness, as caliper, but they fail to report porosity, and they often fail to report the driving pressure for a fluid-flow rate they call permeability. In classifying grades of filter media all of the same material of construction, we look to each for the flow-averaged pore diameter and the thickness.

Capacity of a Filter Medium

The capacity of a filter medium is the volume of a stream that can be fed to a unit area before the resistance climbs by a factor of, say, 10. That is, with a constant fluid-driving pressure, capacity refers to the time before the flow rate falls to, say, $1/10$ of the initial rate. Or, with constant-flow filtration, capacity is the volume filtered before the driving pressure must be increased to, say, 10 times greater than the starting pressure.

In either case, we measure the rate at which the medium loses permeability. Empirical filtration laws point to four different mathematical statements that describe rate losses. Identifying which law one encounters provides additional understanding of the mechanism of filtration. Ideally, we want to see cake filtration, where solids are retained on the surface of the medium. That is, the increasing resistance to flow is due only to the increasing thickness of the cake of collected solids. The pores of the filter are not plugged.

The area of the filter medium required for the filtration job at hand depends, of course, on the volumetric flow rate and the viscosity of the process stream and whether we have a batch or continuous stream. In the latter case, we must decide how often we want to install a fresh filter. More specifically, we must consider the velocity of the stream approaching the face of the medium. It is a direct function of the fluid-driving pressure, the difference in pressure between the upstream face and the downstream face. Obviously, we do not want an undue amount of pressure for fear of rupturing the membrane or rushing the fluid through the membrane so fast that microbes or particles will squeeze through the pores.

Configurations of Membrane Filters

Filtration devices fall into two general types, each type consisting of housing with a replaceable filter medium. One type of housing holds a flat-sheet, 293-mm-diameter membrane or perhaps a stack of such membranes. On a smaller scale, discs are available with diameters as small as 13 mm, along with housings to hold them.

One type of housing is designed to hold cylindrical cartridges, which come in various diameters and lengths, typically about 6.4 cm (2.5 in.) in diameter by 25 cm (10 in.). Each cartridge contains a membrane that is pleated so that a large membrane area — 4000 cm^2 for the 10-inch cartridge — is contained in a relatively small space. Different sized housings hold different numbers of cartridges. Some cartridges contain bundles of hollow fibers, the walls of which constitute the filter medium.

Cross-Flow Filtration

When particles or gels in a stream could quickly clog a membrane, the feed stream is passed across the membrane at high velocity so that solids suspended above the membrane are swept away while clear fluid passes through. The stream flowing across the top of the membrane, called the concentrate, may be returned to the feed tank.

Fibrous Filter Media

Felts of asbestos fibers were formally used as sterilizing filters; one company offered potassium titanate fibers mixed with resin-bound cellulose fibers. Such filters are no longer used as final filters for fear that some fibers may appear in the filtrate. The day may come when small-diameter but long fibers, like the new nanofibers, are used to build a mat that does not release fibers. But until then, fibrous media are only used to prefilter liquids that, in the end, are sterilized and made fiber free by passing through a membrane.

Mats of ordinary-diameter fibers are useful, though, in sterilizing gas streams without release of fibers into the filtrate. Particles and microbes are more easily separated from a gas than from a liquid because of the lower viscosity of gasses. But fibrous media that sterilize gas streams lack small enough pores to pass a bubble-point test. All we have for testing the integrity of a fibrous gas filter is a measure of the gas flow vs. driving pressure. The manufacturer demonstrates that such a filter can stop of cloud of airborne particles or droplets with small diameters. Such filters are employed to clean air fed to fermenters.

The Vent Filter

To be really sure that a gas is sterile, membranes are used. The vent filter cartridge, placed above a tank of liquid, is composed of a hydrophobic membrane. The cartridge allows sterile air to breath into or out of the vessel as the volume of liquid changes, so that the vessel will neither rupture from high pressure nor collapse from low pressure. Because the pores in the vent filter must be small enough to prevent the passage of microbes, water vapor cannot be allowed to condense in the pores. If water vapor did condense there, the differential pressure across the membrane required to blow water from the pores and let air through would be greater than the differential pressure we could allow across the vessel. So a steam jacket is used to keep the vent filter warm enough to prevent condensation.

To determine the area of the membrane surface required for a vent filter, that is, the volumetric flow of air that it must serve, consider the volumetric flow rate of the liquid that will enter or exit the vessel. Thus, before installing a vent cartridge of a certain size or two or more cartridges, look at the specifications around such cartridges in terms of the volumetric flow rate of air it can best handle. As a safety feature, the vessel will be fitted with a pressure-rupture disc.

Gas Filter vs. Liquid Filter

As a rule, a liquid filter meant for sterilization must not be in service for more than one 8-hour shift because a single microbe might pass through the membrane and develop into a colony on the downstream face. If a liquid filter is to be used again for another run, it must be resterilized and retested for integrity. However, during the first run, the membrane may collect enough particles and organic debris to plug some of the pores, in which case the cartridge must be discarded. A vent filter, on the other hand, handles a relatively clean stream; thus, the pores do not readily plug with debris. And a vent filter can be repeatedly steam sterilized and reused. In the manufacturing of antibiotics, vent filters atop fermentation tanks are resteamed as many as 50 times between runs (Meltzer 1987).

The integrity test cannot be performed while the vent filter cartridge is in the process housing. The cartridge must be separately tested in test housing.

The hydrophobic vent cartridge should be soaked in a solution of 50% isopropanol in water to wet and fill the pores. Then follow the pressure hold test and the bubble-point test, understanding that the bubble point is a function of the surface tension of the liquid in the pores. Since isopropanol has a lower surface tension than water, the required bubble-point value (pressure) with the alcohol solution is lower than with pure water. After the cartridge passes these tests, place it in an autoclave to sterilize it and drive off the liquid. Then aseptically place it in the vent housing. The housing has already been sterilized.

Alternatively, a hydrophobic cartridge may be tested for integrity by forcing water against the dry membrane, without having to bother with the alcohol. If a high enough pressure of water is required to force the first flow of water through the largest pores, the cartridge passes the integrity test. But this test has yet to become standard.

In the case of liquid filters, the pressure hold test and the bubble-point test are performed in place. That is, after the cartridge is installed in the housing and the assembly is sterilized, some of the liquid to be filtered is run through to fill the pores of the membranes. Downstream from the filter, plumbing is provided so that this first liquid can be discarded or recycled in case the filter fails the integrity test.

Units of Measure

Before the trend of describing units of measure in SI units, writers, in presenting their findings and examples, have employed a wide variety of units (especially with pressure). The following list offers conversion units relevant to subjects in this book.

Pressure

$N/m^2 = Pa$ (N = Newton, Pa = Pascal)

$1\ lbf/in^2 = 1\ psi = 6.895\ kPa = 144\ lbf/ft^2$

$1\ mm\ Hg = 133\ Pa = 1\ torr$

$1\ cm\ Hg = 1.333\ kPa$

1 inch water = 249 Pa

$1\ atm = 1.013{\cdot}10^5\ Pa = 1.013{\cdot}10^6\ Baryes$, or $dyn/cm^2 = 14.7\ psi$

$1\ bar = 10^6\ Baryes = 0.9869\ atm$

Viscosity

$$1\ centipoise\ (cP) = 10^{-3}\ N{\cdot}s/m^2 = 10^{-3}\ Pa{\cdot}s$$
$$= 10^{-3}\ kg/m{\cdot}s = 2.89\ lbf{\cdot}sec/ft^2$$

$$v = \eta/\rho = 0.22t - 180/t$$

where

v = kinematic viscosity, centistokes
η = absolute viscosity, centipoise
ρ = density, specific gravity
t = Saybolt Universal, seconds

Density

$$1\ \text{g/cc} = 1\ \text{Sp.gr.} = 62.43\ \text{lbm/ft}^3 = 8.34\ \text{lbm/U.S. gal}$$
$$= 1\ \text{kg/liter} = 10^3\ \text{kg/m}^3$$
$$°\text{Bé} = 145 - (145/\text{Sp.gr}),\ \text{for Sp.gr. greater than 1.0.}$$
$$= (140/\text{Sp.gr.}) - 130,\ \text{for Sp.gr. of 1.0 and less.}$$
$$\text{API} = (141.5/\text{Sp.gr.}) - 131.5$$

Surface Tension

$$1\ \text{dyn/cm} = 10^{-3}\text{N/m}$$

Volumetric Flow Rate

$$1\ \text{U.S. gal/min} = 6.31 \cdot 10^{-5}\text{m}^3/\text{s}$$
$$1\ \text{liter/min} = 1.67 \cdot 10^{-5}\ \text{m}^3/\text{s}$$
$$1\ \text{ft}^3/\text{min} = 4.72 \cdot 10^{-5}\ \text{m}^3/\text{s}$$

Area

$$1\ \text{in}^2 = 6.45 \cdot 10^{-4}\ \text{m}^2$$
$$1\ \text{ft}^2 = 9.29 \cdot 10^{-2}\ \text{m}^2$$
$$1\ \text{cm}^2 = 10^{-4}\ \text{m}^2$$

Prefixes

$$\text{M} = \text{mega},\ 10^6$$
$$\text{k} = \text{kilo},\ 10^3$$

c = centi, 10^{-2}

m = milli, 10^{-3} (mm = millimeter)

μ = micro, 10^{-6} (μm = micrometer, old micron)

n = nano, 10^{-9}

Table of Contents

Chapter 10   Filtering Gasses

Chapter 11   The Rating of a Membrane Filter Medium

Chapter 12   Cross-Flow Filtration

Chapter 13   Capacity of a Filter Medium in Constant-Pressure Filtration

1

Liquid Flow through Filter Media

1.1 Overview

Probably the first thing one wants to know about a filter medium meant to clarify a liquid is the relationship between the flow rate of particle-free liquid and the driving pressure. Sometimes the supplier of the medium offers this information. Sometimes one must determine it in order to know what the area of the filter medium should be for the volumetric-flow rate of the stream to be clarified. When the filter medium is a flat sheet, one of the simplest setups to take these measurements involves mounting a small-diameter disk of the medium under a column of clear water and measuring the flow rate. Relate the height of the column to driving pressure.

When the filter medium is larger or in the form of a cartridge, a pump is usually involved along with a suitable housing, a flow meter, and pressure gauges on either side of the housing. Frequently, the exit stream simply discharges at atmospheric pressure (zero gauge pressure). In that case, the pressure drop across the housing, the driving pressure, corresponds to the gauge reading on the feed-stream side. But be sure to measure the pressure-drop across the cartridge alone. Do not include the pressure drop across the housing. Begin by flowing the liquid through the empty housing at different flow rates and recording the various pressure drops. Then, with the filter medium in place, and for different flow rates, subtract the empty-housing pressure drops from the pressure drops read with the medium in place, to obtain the pressure drop across the medium alone.

Having thus measured the liquid-flow rate as a function of driving pressure at three or more driving pressures, plot the data pairs on log/log paper. Or instead of making a plot, simply look to see if the ratios are constant. It does not matter what units of measure are employed. If the ratios are constant, if the points define a straight line with a slope of 1.0, as illustrated by the left portion of Figure 1.1, then the measurements were taken in that range where the ratio of flow rate to driving pressure is constant.

If the slope is less than 1.0, as illustrated by the right portion of Figure 1.1, too much pressure has been applied. Take more measurements at lower

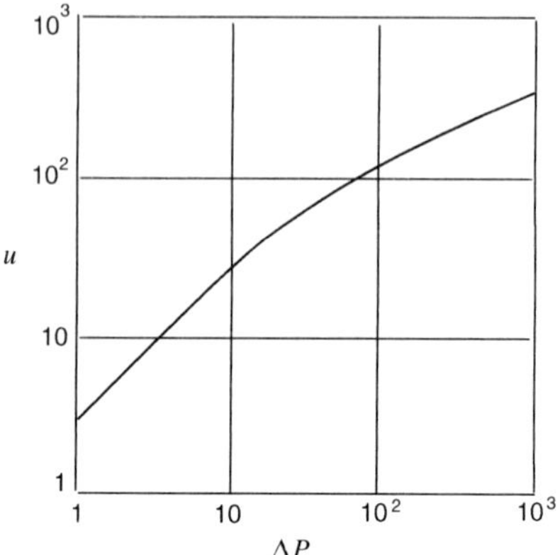

FIGURE 1.1
Example of a plot, on log/log paper, of the velocity, u, with which a liquid approaches the face of a filter medium, vs. the driving pressure, the pressure drop across the two faces, ΔP. The units of measure are arbitrary, but show the slopes described by Equation 1.1. How fast the slope drops from 1.0 to 0.5 is described by Equation 1.2. In filtration, employ the range where the slope is 1.0.

driving pressures (and corresponding lower flow rates). As a rule of thumb in filtration, employ a liquid-approach velocity near 1 gal/min per ft², or 0.0073 m/s. However, in the case of deep-bed filters — for example, a column of sand — the approach velocity may be much greater. Filtration efficiency is a function of fluid residence time in the medium; it increases with increasing residence time.

When the filter medium contains very small pores, make sure the liquid is clear enough so that the medium does not plug with solids during the test. Start by imposing a low driving pressure. After subsequent tests at higher pressures, return to the low pressure, to see if the original flow rate is repeated.

1.2   Understanding the Plot

Recall, approach velocity, $u = Q/A =$ [volumetric flow rate]/[area of the medium]. The plot of Figure 1.1 (Green and Duwez 1951), is described by

$$\frac{\Delta P}{z} = \alpha\eta u + \beta\rho u^2 \tag{1.1}$$

where
$\quad \Delta P =$ the differential pressure, N/m²

z = thickness of the medium, m
α = viscous-term coefficient, m^{-2}
η = absolute viscosity of the liquid, N·s/m^2
β = inertia-term coefficient, m^{-1}
ρ = density of the liquid, kg/m^{2}g$_c$ (g$_c$ = 1 kg·m/N·s^2)

While Equation 1.1 suggests plotting ΔP on the vertical axis in Figure 1.1, it is plotted as shown for later discussions. The line of Figure 1.1 changes slope from 1.0 to 0.5 at the rate defined by Green and Duwez (1951).

$$f = 2/Re + 2 \tag{1.2}$$

where
f = friction factor = $(2\Delta P/z)/\beta\rho u^2$ = (total forces)/(half inertia forces)
Re = Reynolds number = $\beta\rho u/\alpha\eta$ = (inertia forces)/(viscous forces)

1.3 Separating Viscous Flow from Inertia Flow

In Figure 1.1, the slope of 1.0 indicates viscous (laminar) flow. Viscous drag is the predominate resistance to flow. At higher velocities, the slope falls to 0.5, as inertia flow predominates. The liquid is changing direction so fast that viscous drag has been eclipsed. Where the slope is changing and, indeed, when much of the resistance to flow lies with inertia, the flow of liquid is still laminar (Rosenstein et al. 1980). It is not turbulent, as some writers have surmised; indeed, the Reynolds number in Equation 1.2 has not exceeded single digits. Turbulent flow in a pipe is associated with Reynolds numbers greater than 3000. Interestingly enough, when a single fiber is held in a stream, eddy currents develop around it, but around a fibrous mat, no such eddy currents appear.

Given the data of Figure 1.1, deduce the values of α and β in Equation 1.1 by making a plot (not shown here) of $\Delta P/zu$ vs. u to define the line

$$\frac{\Delta P}{zu} = \alpha\eta + \beta\rho u \tag{1.3}$$

where the intercept is $\alpha\eta$ and the slope is $\beta\rho$.

The ratio β/α is not the same from one medium to another (Green and Duwez 1951). But, assigning a meaning to β, other than calling it the inertia-term coefficient, is not important because filtration is performed at velocities where the second term of Equation 1.1 is nil. Values of β are smaller than α. But, of course, a dense liquid (such as carbon tetrachloride), with a high value of ρ, will increase the magnitude of the inertia term. Sometimes, as in the case of pleated-paper filter cartridges, where the area of the filter medium is not known, one must plot volumetric flow rate (rather than approach velocity) vs. driving pressure, to find the region where the slope is 1.0. Again, do not include the pressure drop across the housing.

1.4   The Meaning of Permeability

The data presented above regarding the ratios of flow rate to driving pressure will obviously be different for a liquid of another viscosity. Thus, to characterize a filter medium for any liquid, deduce the viscous permeability of the medium. It is important to understand this term, because it is a basic characteristic of a filter medium and it is used in deducing the flow-averaged pore size.

In the case of a flat-sheet medium where the liquid flow is directly proportional to the driving force (the slope is 1.0 in the Figure 1.1 kind of plot), deduce viscous permeability, B (m^2), from

$$B = \frac{1}{\alpha} = \frac{u\eta z}{\Delta P} = \frac{Q\eta z}{A\Delta P} \tag{1.4}$$

where
 Q = volumetric flow rate of liquid, m^3/s
 A = area of the filter medium, m^2

The other terms were defined with Equation 1.1.

When the filter medium is a thick-walled tube or candle of outside radius r_1, inside radius r_2, and length L, and liquid flows from the outside wall to the inside wall, calculate permeability from

$$B = \frac{Q\eta \ln(r_1/r_2)}{\Delta P 2\pi L} \tag{1.5}$$

where *ln* indicates natural logarithm (Johnston 1982a).

However, do not take permeability measurements with a long cartridge. How long is long? Perhaps longer than 5 inches. Flows through the walls are not uniform. The measurements are distorted by the pressure drop along the length of the inner diameter and of the hydrostatic head. One would think that someone would have already addressed this subject, but this writer has yet to see even a theoretical study.

Previous writers have expressed permeability in darcies. The conversion to SI units is: 1 darcy = 0.987·10^{-12}m^2, since, by definition, B, in Equation 1.4, equals one darcy when

$$Q = 1 \text{ cc/s} = 10^{-6} \text{m}^3/\text{s}$$
$$A = 1 \text{ cm}^2 = 10^{-4} \text{m}^2$$
$$\eta = 1 \text{ centipoise} = 10^{-3} \text{N·s/m}^2$$
$$z = 1 \text{ cm} = 10^{-2} \text{m}$$
$$\Delta P = 1 \text{ atmosphere} = 1.103 \cdot 10^5 \text{N/m}^2$$

1.5   Concepts of Pore Size

Before describing how to deduce the flow-averaged pore size, consider what it is we think we are measuring. The key to a direct understanding of pore size lies in examining that singular product, the track-etched membrane. It contains neat, circular holes (pores) going straight through it. Thus, we can describe a pore as having a certain diameter and a certain length. And, for the most part, all the pores have the same diameter and length, the latter being equal to the thickness of the membrane, usually 10 µm. Occasionally, two or more holes are crowded together to make one larger opening. About 10% of the membrane surface constitutes the cross-sectional area of the pores. Described in three-dimensional terms, 10% of the bulk volume of the membrane is void space; i.e., the porosity of the membrane, ε, is 0.10.

1.6   Complicated Pore Geometry

On examining a sponge-like, microporous membrane, manufactured by the solvent-cast method, we see the porosity to be near 0.7–0.8. In addressing the diameter of an irregularly shaped pore on the surface, we consider the ratio of cross-sectional area to perimeter, called the hydraulic diameter. And we see a relatively broad distribution of pore diameters. Further, microporous membranes are about 15 times as thick as a track-etched membrane. So while we can easily speak of the average pore size in the track-etched membrane as being the size of one of the many same-sized pores, we realize that with the microporous membrane we must consider the meaning of an average pore size.

The same reasoning holds for fibrous mats, which also have porosities near 0.8, with greater porosities for the filtration of gases. But there's more. As we consider fluid flow through these media — defining different tunnels — we realize that within each tunnel the diameter varies along the length. And different tunnels have different lengths. The average tunnel length is greater than the thickness of the medium. Thus, to speak of an average pore size we must consider the average of many distributions.

When the filter medium is a bed of granules, we have the same problem in defining pore size as we have with the microporous membranes and fibrous mats. Further, the problem of deducing an average pore size grows more complex when the porosity of the bed changes with depth. Indeed, ordinary filter paper has a greater packing density of fibers on one face. The machine-forming wire side is denser than the other face. And thick-walled, tubular cartridges often have differences in densities across the thickness of the walls.

1.7 Pore Size and Porosity

By building a filter medium by packing given-sized granules or fibers closer together, thus reducing the porosity of the filter medium, we decrease the diameter of the average-sized pore. In addition, while we can build fibrous beds with a broad range of porosities, we cannot do so with granules. If the granules are too far apart, they cannot stick together. Filter media built of granules usually fall into a porosity range of about 0.2 to 0.4.

1.8 Different Kinds of Average Pore Diameters

In considering a pore-size distribution, and the corresponding average pore size, we must decide which of the following three distributions to address (Chapter 3 discusses pore-size distributions in more detail):

- In the number distribution, we consider a list of the counts of pores of different diameters seen in a thin plane of the medium.

- In the volume distribution, the cross-sectional opening is said to have unit depth, and thus the volume of a pore is proportional to the square of the diameter.

- When a fluid, in viscous flow (see Section 1.9), under a given driving force, confronts a pore, the volumetric flow rate of the fluid through the pore is proportional to the square of the cross-sectional area.

Thus, the flow-averaged pore diameter is larger than the volume-averaged, which, in turn, is larger than the number-averaged. Yet, some writers say the volume-distribution of pore diameters is the same as the fluid-flow distribution. And, many writers report pore size without explaining what they mean, radius or diameter, or how they measured it.

1.9 Deducing the Flow-Averaged Pore Diameter

Recall the Hagen-Poiseuille Law for viscous flow of fluid through a tube: For a fluid of viscosity η, the average velocity u, of the fluid is related to the tube diameter d, and pressure drop ΔP, along a length z as

$$\frac{d^2}{32} = \frac{u\eta z}{\Delta P} \tag{1.6}$$

Now employ Equation 1.6 to reach a measurement of the averaged pore diameter defined by liquid flow. We realize that the average velocity of the liquid within the medium is the ratio of the approach velocity to the porosity, u/ε. And the average pore length is the thickness times the tortuosity factor, $z\tau$. When the building blocks of a filter medium are arrayed in a random manner, $\tau = 1/\varepsilon$, deduced as follows (ASTM F902).

Imagine a plane in a filter medium perpendicular to the flow of fluid. On this plane we draw a grid where the size of a single square in the grid corresponds to the size of the flow-averaged pore. Consider that this grid has a thickness corresponding to the length of the sides of the square grid. That is, we have a plane of cubes: some empty (the pores); some filled (the filter medium).

Now consider slugs of fluid approaching the medium. The probability, p, that a cube is empty corresponds to the porosity. The probability that a cube is occupied (solid) is q, equal to $1-p$. Consider that N slugs of fluid approach this grid, and the size of a slug corresponds to the size of a cube. We expect that Np slugs will pass straight through the grid. That is, the distance traveled through the grid equals the thickness.

Of those Nq slugs that hit a solid cube, and have to take a single side step, Npq slugs find an empty cube, and Nq^2 do not. The total distance traveled by the Npq slugs in passing through the grid is thus twice the thickness. Of those Nq^2 slugs still on the grid, Npq^2 find an empty cube after two side steps and thus travel a distance of three times the thickness of the grid in passing through. Continuing with this logic, the average distance traveled by all slugs, as a multiple of the grid thickness, the tortuosity factor, is

$$\tau = \frac{N(p + 2pq + 2pq^2 + 4pq^3 ...)}{N} = \frac{1}{p} = \frac{1}{\varepsilon} \tag{1.7}$$

Thus, from Equation 1.6 and Equation 1.7, deduce the flow-averaged pore diameter, d_{av}, via

$$(d_{av})^2 = \frac{32u\eta\tau}{\Delta P\varepsilon} = \frac{32B\tau}{\varepsilon} = \frac{32B}{\varepsilon^2} \tag{1.8}$$

In a woven cloth, the value of τ lies between 1.0 and $1/\varepsilon$. Employing Equation 1.8 assumes that the liquid employed does not swell the materials of the filter medium and thereby change the porosity and (or) the thickness. If swelling is suspected, separately deduce permeability via gas flow, addressed in Chapter 2.

1.10 The Streaming Potential

As a fluid flows through a porous material, a voltage drop develops between the fluids on the two different sides of the porous material. When the fluid is flammable it becomes important to ground both fluids to avoid sparks and subsequent fire or explosion.

The streaming potential is also of interest in water filtration since it provides an indication of the zeta potential of the medium. Particles in a feed stream also carry a zeta potential, and filtration efficiency is a function of how well the pore walls of the filter medium attract or repel the particles, depending in differences in zeta potentials of the walls and the particles.

To measure the streaming potential of a filter medium in water flow, employ an all-plastic housing fitted with reference electrodes (such as silver/ silver chloride) close to the separate faces of the filter medium. Connect the electrodes to an electrometer, which measures voltage while drawing a minimum amount of current. Collect data to make the plot, on linear/linear coordinates, of streaming potential, E (vertical axis), vs. pressure drop, ΔP (not fluid-flow rate). Oulman and Baumann (1970) discuss the details of this analysis.

Often it is not necessary to calculate the absolute value of the zeta potential. That is, it is sufficient to examine the direction of and magnitude of the slope of the plot of E vs. ΔP, while considering the following points (Bocquet 1951; Worthy 1984):

- Positive slope indicates a positive zeta potential (and a negative slope indicates negative potential). In some cases all one wants to know is the sign of the potential.

- Direction of the electric current wanting to flow through the filter medium is the same as the direction of fluid flow; hence, the cathode is the electrode under higher pressure (on the feed face of the filter medium).

- The resulting streaming potential rising out of the liquid-flow rate is independent of the geometry of the filter medium. It depends on the material of construction and, apparently, on the surface area of the pore walls washed by a unit volume of fluid.

- Using metal electrodes, water can be made to flow through a porous material by imposing electric power instead of driving pressure, as in the dewatering of clay (Yukawa 1971).

1.11 Compatibility of Different Liquids with Different Filter Media

Microporous filter membranes are built of different polymers. Table 1.1 provides a summary of compatibility data.

TABLE 1.1

Compatibility of Membrane Filters

Membrane Material	General Use	Limitations
Cellulose esters	Aqueous solutions	Alcohols, proteins, DMF[a], strong acids and bases
Polysulfone	Proteinaceous and aqueous solutions	Benzyl alcohol and DMF
Polyvinylidene diflouride	Same as above	Acetone, DMF, strong acids and bases
Nylon 66	Aqueous and solvent solutions	Conc. NaOH, proteins, formic and hydrofluoric acids
Nylon with positive charge	Aqueous solutions	Same as Nylon 66
Nylon hydroxyl modified	Proteinaceous solutions	None
Polycarbonate	Aqueous solutions	None[b]
Polytetra-fluoroethylene	Air, solvents	Hydrophobic[c]

[a] Dimethylformamide.

[b] Some users avoid the track-etched membrane, $^1/_{10}$ the thickness of other membranes, and with a porosity of 0.1, instead of 0.8, feeling that the occasional, extra-large, straight-through pores will let microbes through.

[c] At least one supplier offers a hydrophilic type.

Source: Modified from McKinnon and Avis (1993).

2

Gas Flow through Filter Media

2.1 Introduction

A common gas-flow test for filter papers and nonwoven cloths is called the Frazier, in which an upstream air gauge pressure of 0.5 lbf/in^2 (psi) is applied to a 2-inch diameter disk of the filter medium as the downstream face is exposed to the atmosphere (0 gauge pressure). The airflow from the downstream face is reported as ft^3/min·ft^2. Some writers have referred to that measurement as permeability. Alternatively, the resistance is reported, say, in mm of water, to an approach velocity of, say, 10.5 ft/min. In these tests the investigator assumes he or she is in the viscous flow range: that range where the ratio of flow rate to driving pressure is constant for somewhat smaller and larger driving pressures. Setups for panel filters are described in ASTM F778.

When the absolute gas pressure (gauge pressure plus atmospheric pressure) on the upstream face of a filter medium is not greater than 1.1 times the absolute pressure on the downstream face, and when the rated pore diameters are larger than about 1 µm, then Equation 1.1, in liquid flow, can apply. Also Equation 1.4 and Equation 1.5 can be used to deduce the permeability, and Equation 1.8 can be used to deduce the flow-averaged pore diameter. But when the differential pressure is higher, or when rated pore diameters are smaller than about 1 µm, two other equations are required to describe gas flow. And a different kind of plot is made to relate gas velocity to driving pressure.

To perform a gas-flow test with a flat sheet filter medium, it is convenient to expose the downstream face to the atmosphere, so we know that the absolute pressure there is one atmosphere. Place the upstream tap for the pressure gauge directly over the upstream face of the medium. Employ a mass-flow meter (such as a rota- or float meter) in the upstream line. Such meters are usually calibrated to read volumetric flow rate at atmospheric pressure. With increasing pressures on the upstream face, record the corresponding increases in gas flow.

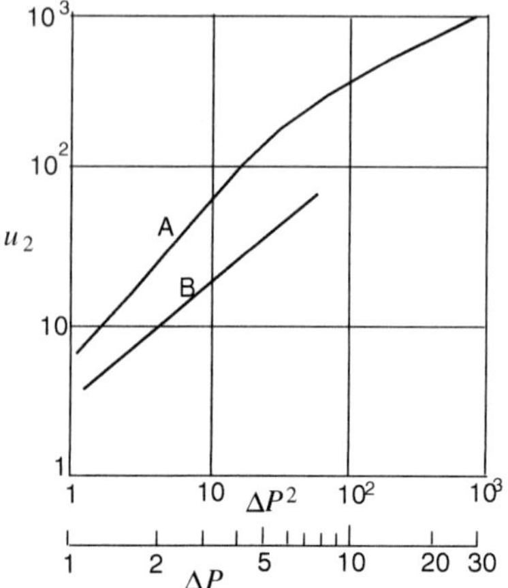

FIGURE 2.1

Examples of gas-flow measurements through filter membranes. Units of measure are arbitrary but show the shapes of lines seen in plots on log/log paper of the volumetric velocity of gas leaving the low-pressure face, u_2, as a function of the pressure drops, ΔP, across the two faces. The ΔP scale is shown for discussion in Chapter 4. Of interest here is the ΔP^2 scale showing that Line A, with an initial slope of 1.0 against ΔP^2, falls to 0.5 as inertia forces overwhelm viscous drag, following Equation 2.1, but only for membranes with *rated* pore diameters larger than about 0.5 μm. Line B is seen with rated pore diameters smaller than about 0.5 μm, with slopes less than 1.0, depending of the amount of Knudsen flow diluting viscous flow. Apparently inertia flow is not reached.

Before making the plot we are about to describe, convert the flow rate to the volumetric velocity of the gas leaving the downstream face — if you know the surface area. If the surface area is unknown, simply record the volumetric flow rate of the emerging gas. On log/log paper, make a plot of the downstream velocity, u_2 (or downstream volumetric flow rate) vs. the square of the driving pressure, ΔP^2, as shown in Figure 2.1 (Green and Duwez 1951).

For filter media rated as having pore diameters larger than about 1 μm, the plot will look like Curve A. That is, the line starts out with a slope of 1.0, against the ΔP^2 scale, in viscous flow, then falls to 0.5 in inertia flow. The ΔP scale is shown for discussion in Chapter 4. For filter media with rated pore diameters smaller than about 0.5 μm, the plot will look like Line B. That is, the line remains straight; however, the slope lies between 0.5 and 1.0. Line B shows a combination of viscous flow and Knudsen flow (diffusion flow, sometimes called slip flow). Apparently, inertia flow is not reached (Badenhop 1983).

As in the case of liquid flow tests, be sure the pressure-drop measurements across the medium do not include pressure drops across the housing. Further, remember that even if the feed-stream pressure is high (as in a compressed-air line) and the filtrate pressure is also high, the items of interest are the differential pressure and the corresponding volumetric flow rate from the downstream face. When the filter medium is soft, high differential pressures may compress the medium, reducing its porosity, making it, in effect, a different medium.

2.2 Filters with Rated Pore Diameters Larger than 0.5 μm

Consider Curve A in Figure 2.1 where the slope starts out as 1.0, against the ΔP^2 scale, then drops to 0.5. In such a filter medium, the description of gas flow is written as

$$\frac{(\Delta P)^2}{z} = \alpha \eta P_2 u_2 + \frac{\beta \left(P_2 u_2\right)^2 M}{R g_c T} \tag{2.1}$$

where

ΔP = absolute pressure on the upstream face, P_1, minus that on the downstream face, P_2, N/m^2
z = thickness of the medium, m
α = the viscous term coefficient m^{-2}
η = absolute viscosity of the gas, N·s/m^2
β = the inertia-term coefficient, m^{-1}
u_2 = velocity of gas leaving the downstream face, at P_2, m/s
M = molecular weight of the gas, kg/mole
R = gas constant, 5314 N·m/mole·T
T = absolute temperature, K (°C + 273)
g_c = conversion constant, 1 kg·m/N·s^2

As in liquid filtration, the rate at which the slope changes is described by Equation 1.2. And, as in liquid filtration, our interest lies with the slope-equals-1.0 portion of Curve A, when the second term of Equation 2.1 is nil. That is, permeability, B, equals $1/\alpha$, and, if we know the porosity, ε, we can deduce the flow-averaged pore diameter via Equation 1.8.

2.3 Filters with Rated Pore Diameters Smaller than 0.5 μm

If the gas-flow plot looks like Line B in Figure 2.1, we cannot deduce the viscous-flow-averaged pore diameter from gas-flow data, because viscous flow is diluted with Knudsen (diffusion) flow. To deduce which portions of the flow are viscous and which are Knudsen, drop the inertia term of Equation 2.1 and replace it with a slip-flow term. That is, drop the second term in Equation 2.1, rearrange the equation, then add a second term to obtain

$$u_2 = \frac{\Delta P^2}{z\alpha\eta P_2} + \frac{S\Delta P}{zP_2} \tag{2.2}$$

where S is the gas diffusion rate, m^2/s, a function of the molecular weight and temperature of the gas and of the diameters of the pores. The smaller the diameters, the more diffusion, the more slip flow.

To deduce which portion of the flow is viscous, and which portion is diffusion, rearrange Equation 2.2 to obtain

$$\frac{u_2 P_2 z}{\Delta P} = \frac{P_{av}}{\alpha\eta} + S \tag{2.3}$$

Following that equation, make a plot on linear/linear coordinates as illustrated in Figure 2.2. In that figure the top line shows total flow, while the bottom line shows viscous flow. That is, viscous flow is drawn with the same slope as the total flow, but shows zero viscous flow when pressures on both faces of the medium are equal, that is, when $P_{av} = (P_1 + P_2)/2 =$ one atmosphere. For a more detailed discussion of S, see Badenhop (1983), Carman (1956), Scheidegger (1963), and Treybal (1980).

In general, S, Knudsen flow, in a capillary tube of diameter d is a function of d^2, rather than d^4, as in viscous (Hagen-Poiseuille) flow. We keep these facts in mind when in Chapter 4 we discuss the extended bubble-point test as a way of measuring the pore size distribution on the faces of microporous membranes.

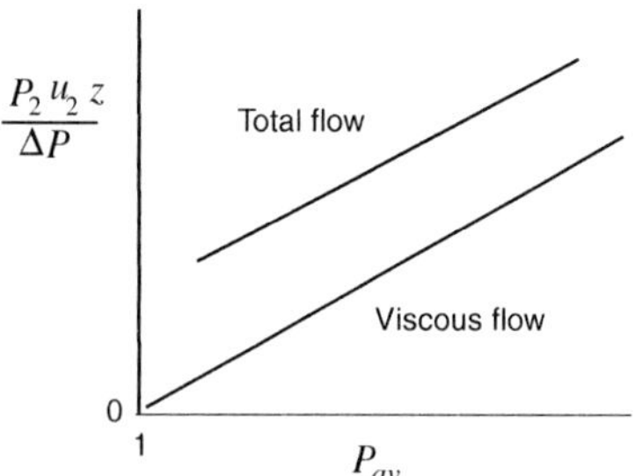

FIGURE 2.2

Example of plots on linear/linear coordinates via Equation 2.3 of gas flow through filter membranes with rated pore diameters smaller than about 0.5 μm. From the total-flow line, indicating both viscous and Knudsen flow, draw a parallel line passing through the origin to show the portion of flow that is viscous. Where P_{av} is 1.0 atmosphere, ΔP is zero; hence no viscous flow occurs.

2.4 Examples of Gas-Slip Flow Comparison to Liquid-Viscous Flow

When measuring fluid flow rates through a filter medium with a liquid on the one hand and with a gas on the other, we expect to see the same values of permeability. But where the pores are small, and slip flow occurs (and we are not aware that it does), the deduced value of permeability (and the flow-averaged pore size) will be larger with the gas-flow measurements.

Consider, in Figure 2.3, data from Millipore Corporation's Catalogue MC/1. It provides both water- and air-flow rates, under a common driving pressure, through a series of cellulose–ester microporous filter membranes. All the membranes have essentially the same porosity and thickness, but the rated pore diameters differ, ranging from 0.05 to 5.0 μm. While we would expect the velocity of both air and water to decline by the same amount with decreasing pore size — all circles will fall on a line with slope of 1.0 — we

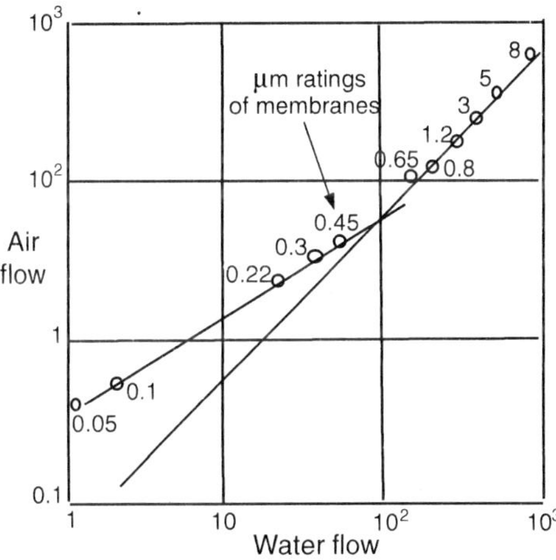

FIGURE 2.3

Illustrations of gas-slip flow as a function of the rated pore diameters in microporous filter membranes. The vertical axis shows air flow from the downstream face, L/min·cm², from a gauge pressure on the upstream face at 13.5 psi, vs. water flow, on the horizontal axis, from the downstream face, mL/min·cm², at the same driving pressure. Membranes vary in rated pore diameters but are of equal thickness and porosity. From *rated* pore diameters of 8.0 μm down to near 0.5 μm, the correlation line follows a slope of 1.0. Below those ratings, air flows depart from viscous flow with the addition of Knudsen flows. The smaller the pores, the more Knudsen flows. Some investigators have measured the air permeability of microporous membranes or beds of fine particles without considering the possibility of Knudsen flow. (Plotted from data in Millipore Catalogue MC/1 1971.)

see instead that below a certain rated pore diameter, the velocity of air does not fall as fast as the velocity of water. Below a rated pore diameter near 0.5 μm, the bend in the line, slip flow occurs. And the ratio of slip flow to viscous flow increases with smaller pores. The rated pore diameter is an arbitrary assignment, addressed in Chapter 11.

2.5   Comparing Liquid Flow to Gas Flow

Suppose a filter medium shows the symptoms of viscous flow with both a gas and a liquid, and we have measured the porosity. In this case, our deduction of the flow-averaged pore diameter should be the same for both fluids. But, suppose our calculations indicate a smaller flow-averaged pore diameter value with liquid flow than for gas flow, and we are sure that no gas flow is due to to slip flow. Further, we are sure that in the liquid-flow test the liquid did not contain enough solids to partially fill, or blind, the pores. In such cases it is apparent that the liquid swells the building blocks of the filter medium.

3

The Most Probable Pore-Size Distribution

3.1 Modeling Random Pore-Size Distributions

Before addressing fluid intrusion studies as a way of characterizing filter media and deducing pore-size distributions, let us consider one mechanical model and two mathematical models of random pore-size distributions. The structure of a track-etched membrane is simple. Using high-energy radiation followed by leaching of the damaged tracks, a 10-µm-thick polycarbonate film is drilled with round holes that go straight through. Since the holes are located randomly, the porosity, the ratio of open areas to bulk area, is kept at only 10%. (The diameters of the pores are a function of the leaching time.) Placing more pores would result in overlap, making some extra large pores. Thus, the vast majority of the pores have the same diameter; the pore-size distributions are very narrow. But because the permeabilities of such membranes are low, they are only used for analytical filtration where investigators want to be sure that particles or microbes larger than a certain size are captured.

Commercial fine filtration is done with thicker (150-µm) membranes with porosities near 70 to 80% and thus greater permeabilities. Such membranes, produced by the solvent-cast method, are essentially sponge-like with a random array of pores of different sizes. Similarly, mats of nonwoven fibers and sheets of sintered granules with random arrays of materials also contain random pore-size distributions. Imagine slicing a thin layer from the surface of one of these commercial filter media, so thin we can see straight through the pores. We see an array of openings of different shapes and sizes. We define the diameter of a pore as the ratio of the cross-sectional area to the perimeter (the hydraulic diameter). We then make a list of the numbers of pores of different diameters. What sort of a pore-size distribution do we expect to see?

Piekaar and Clarenburg (1967) provide an answer. They randomly drew short lines of different slopes on a plane, as if dropping toothpicks on a surface, thus defining polygons of various sizes. They measured the cross-sectional area of each polygon as well as its perimeter and calculated the

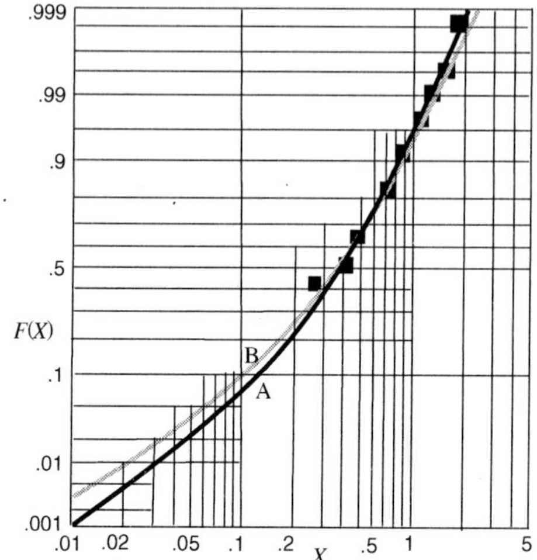

FIGURE 3.1

Cumulative numbers of pores, $F(X)$, of X diameters, in a thin layers of a filter medium, according to Math Model A (Equation 3.4), Model B (Equation 3.6), and the points of Piekaar and Clarenburg (1967).

diameters of pores from the ratios of areas to perimeters. On log-probability paper, they plotted the cumulative numbers of pores vs. diameter, as illustrated by the points in Figure 3.1. Believing that their points must be part of a straight line, they concluded that the distribution is log normal, since a log-normal distribution is a straight line on this kind of plot. Piekaar and Clarenburg (1967) further reported that with more lines (more toothpicks) and more and smaller pores defined, the slope of the line in their plot did not change. That is, the ratio of the geometric standard deviation to the mean did not change with changes in the mean. That ratio remained at 1.9. Curves A and B in Figure 3.1 show the cumulative numbers of pores using two separate math models. That is, the math models show curves instead of straight lines. Because Piekaar and Clarenburg (1967) do not show points below the 40th percentile mark, we cannot say which math model better fits the mechanical model (or vice versa).

3.2   Math Model A

Math Model A is deduced as follows Johnston (1983). Consider a thin layer of a filter medium. The probability that a spot on that layer is part of a pore corresponds to the porosity, ε, the ratio of open area to bulk area. On moving away from that spot for X numbers of unit distances, the probability that the pore has a radius or diameter, X, corresponds to ε^X. Thus, the relative number of pores, N, of diameter X, corresponds to

$$N_X \approx X\varepsilon^X \tag{3.1}$$

Realizing that $\varepsilon^X = e^{X\ln\varepsilon} = \exp(X \ln \varepsilon)$, we replace $\ln \varepsilon$ with β, a scale factor, reflecting the sizes of the solids in the filter medium as well as the packing density. And, since $\ln \varepsilon$ is negative, it follows that the Equation 3.1 can be written as Equation 3.2 (Johnston 1998c).

$$N_X \approx \frac{X}{\exp(\beta X)} \tag{3.2}$$

Equation 3.2 corresponds to the gamma distribution, Equation 3.3.

$$f(X) = \left[\frac{\beta^\alpha}{\Gamma(\alpha)}\right]\frac{X^{\alpha-1}}{\exp(\beta X)} \tag{3.3}$$

where
    α = distribution shape factor
    β = scale factor
    X = pore diameter or radius
    α/β = the arithmetic mean, μ
    $\alpha/\beta^2 = \sigma^2 =$ variance (σ = standard deviation)
    $\sigma/\mu = \alpha^{-0.5*}$
    $\Gamma(\alpha) = (\alpha - 1)!$ Recall that $0! = 1$

The term in brackets is the normalizing factor, providing that the area under the curve is unity (1.0 square X unit). Thus, for the number distribution of pore diameters (or radii), $\alpha = 2$, corresponding to Equation 3.2.

Now consider that in Equation 3.3 the mean, μ, is 0.443 units (for comparison to Math Model B with the same mean). Since $\alpha = 2$ and $\mu = \alpha/\beta = 0.443$, it follows that $\beta = 4.519$. Thus, Equation 3.3 becomes Equation 3.4.

$$f(X) = [20.387]\frac{X}{\exp(4.519X)} \tag{3.4}$$

The cumulative function of Equation 3.4 plots in Figure 3.1 as Curve A. The density function plots in Figure 3.2 also as Curve A.

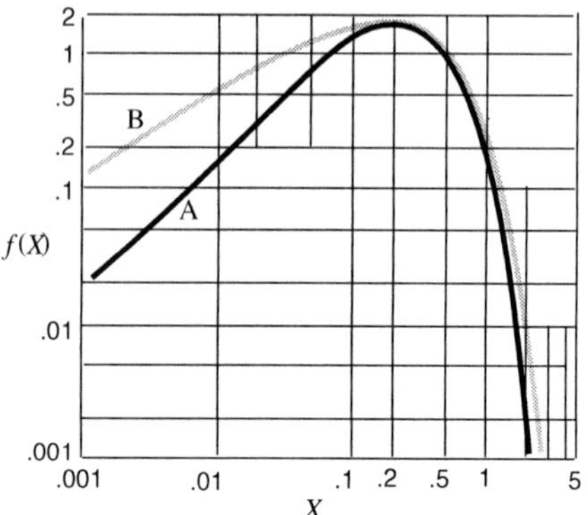

FIGURE 3.2
Curve A, a plot of Equation 3.4; Curve B of Equation 3.6.

3.3   Math Model B

Math Model B, in Figure 3.1 and Figure 3.2, follows a more complicated expression, offered by Corte and Lloyd (1966). They imagine a thin, random array of fibers on a page, as do Piekaar and Clarenburg (1967), who do not cite Corte and Lloyd. Corte and Lloyd approach the probability question by reasoning that the distances between fibers crossing a horizontal line follow a gamma distribution, as do distances crossing a vertical line. It then follows that the distribution of pore areas corresponds to a gamma-squared distribution.

Corte and Lloyd (1966) conclude that the number distribution of pore radii, X, is described by

$$f(X) = X \, Ko(X) \tag{3.5}$$

where Ko is the zeroth order modified Bessel function of the second kind. Unfortunately, when Corte and Lloyd (1966) point to where that function is tabulated they point to a wrong reference. More recently Dodson and Sampson (1966) reviewed the work of Corte and Lloyd, and Dodson graciously provided this writer with a tabulation of that Bessel function, which is plotted in Figure 3.3.

The gamma-squared distribution also contains a distribution-shape factor, k, and a scale factor, b. Of interest in the Dodson and Sampson (1966) review are their Equation 7 and Equation 8 for deducing the mean pore radius, μ, and the variance, σ^2. In those equations, $k = 1.0$ for the number distribution. Thus, with $k = 1$, and with $b = 1$,

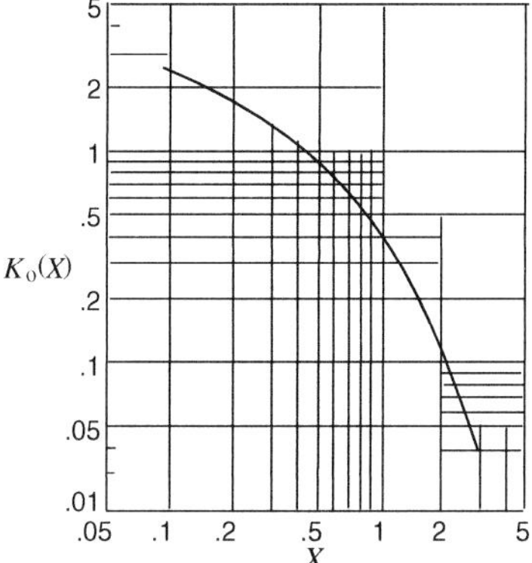

FIGURE 3.3
$Ko(X)$ = values of the zeroth order modified Bessel function of the second kind.

$$\mu = \frac{\sqrt{\pi}}{4} = 0.443$$

$$\sigma = \left[\frac{1}{\pi} - \frac{\pi}{16}\right]^{0.5} = 0.349$$

We then wondered if that distribution could be described by the single-gamma distribution, Equation 3.3. If so the single-gamma function would have the following parameters: $\sigma/\mu = 0.349/0.443 = 0.7878 = \alpha^{-0.5}$, so that $\alpha = 1.61123$; $\mu = \alpha/\beta = 0.443 = 1.61123/\beta$, so that, $\beta = 3.637$.

We thus consider the single-gamma expression

$$f(X) = [8.956]\frac{X^{0.61123}}{\exp(3.637X)} \tag{3.6}$$

Figure 3.2 shows the density-function plot of Equation 3.6, labeled B. That plot, on log/log paper, follows the shape seen in a plot of $X\,Ko(X)$ vs. X, shown by Corte and Lloyd (1966), when we plot their curve on log/log paper. Thus, in this case, the single-gamma distribution does represent the gamma-squared distribution.

Dodson and Sampson (1996), addressing the Bessel function, which they call $Ko(z)$, explain that $z = 2br\pi^{0.5}$, where r = pore radius, and b = the scale factor. The cumulative plot of Equation 3.6 is the B Curve of Figure 3.1.

3.4 Laminar Fluid Flow through These Models

Now let us consider laminar flow of liquid through a thin sheet of pores. Under a given driving pressure, the volumetric flow rate through a tube is proportional to the square of the cross-sectional area, or the diameter, X, of the tube to the 4th power (Hagen-Poiseuille Law). However, flows through orifices, as imagined here, are proportional to only X^2. Nonetheless, Rosenstein et al. (1980) demonstrated that flow through a porous medium *is* laminar. That is, while a single fiber held in a stream develops eddy currents, no such currents develop in a bed of fibers.

Thus, to describe the volumetric flow rate of liquid through the Model-A layer of pores, we write

$$f(X) = [78.5]\frac{X^4}{\exp(4.515X)} \quad \text{Model A} \tag{3.7}$$

And, to describe the volumetric-flow rate through a Model-B layer of pores we write

$$f(X) = [27.31]\frac{X^{2.445}}{\exp(3.637X)} \quad \text{Model B} \tag{3.8}$$

These equations plot as the curves in Figure 3.4.

3.5 Fluid Flow through Many Layers

Now let us consider fluid flow through a stack of layers. Let us also consider, for a moment, that the porosity of all layers is the same. That is, all layers have the same packing density of solids and the same pore-size distribution. But, of course, the location of a certain-size pore in one layer is not necessarily the same as in adjacent layers. So if we consider flow through, say, 10 layers, we modify the above single-layer flows with the following equations.

Model A, 10 layers

$$f(X) = 8.8 \cdot 10^{19}\left(\frac{X^4}{\exp(4.519X)}\right)^{10} \tag{3.9}$$

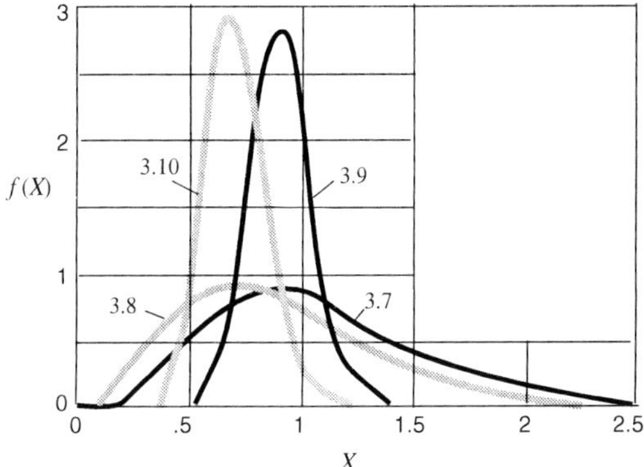

FIGURE 3.4
Plots of various equations.

Model B, 10 Layers

$$f(X) = 2.0 \cdot 10^{15} \left(\frac{X^{2.445}}{\exp(3.671X)} \right)^{10} \tag{3.10}$$

These equations also plot as the distributions in Figure 3.4. We see that as fluid flows through many layers it defines a narrow, symmetrical pore-size distribution, in which the flow-averaged pore size corresponds to the most-popular flow-pore size in a single layer. Further, that overall flow-averaged pore diameter is deduced via Equation 1.8. Yet many filter media have smaller porosities (greater packing densities) on one face than on the other, meaning one face has smaller pores. Thus, when measuring the bubble point, addressed in Chapter 4, the alert investigator will determine the bubble point on the separate faces and will also perform the extended-bubble-point test on both faces. This writer has yet to see the results of such a dual examination.

4

Characterizing Filter Media Using Fluid Intrusion Measurements

4.1 The Bubble Point

In principle, bubble-point measurement is simple. Place a 47-mm-diameter disk of a filter medium into a suitable housing. Flood it with water, making sure all pores are filled, leaving a layer of water on top. From underneath apply a slowly increasing pressure of air. Look for the first perceptible bubble coming out of the water layer. When the bubble appears, note the pressure underneath. That is the bubble point. Deduce the diameter of the largest pores from that pressure and the surface tension of the wetting liquid, as explained in Figure 4.1. In this test, much of the water in the medium is pushed to the top as the largest pores on the surface blow open. More pressure is required to blow open the smaller pores.

When using this method, however, bear in mind that the pores are not cylinders. That is, even if we know the angle with which the liquid wets the inner wall of a tube of the material of the medium, how do we translate that

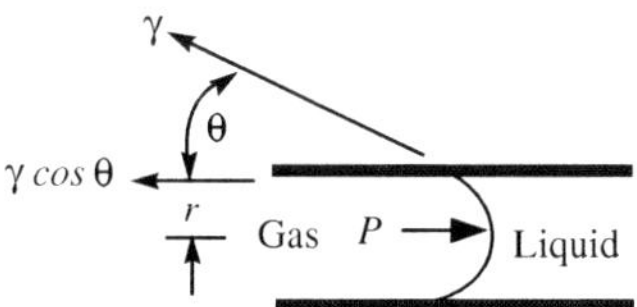

FIGURE 4.1

With a tube of small radius, r, or diameter, d,. gas pressure from the left is resisted by liquid from the right. Liquid wets the walls at a wetting angle θ. The surface tension of the liquid, γ, (N/m) acting along the cosine vector, resists the gas pressure according to

$$P = \frac{perimeter\ force}{area} = \frac{2\pi\gamma\cos\theta}{\pi r^2} = \frac{2\gamma\cos\theta}{r} = \frac{4\gamma\cos\theta}{d}$$

to the rough walls in the medium? And even if we know the surface tension of the liquid used to flood the medium ($72 \cdot 10^{-3}$ N/m for pure water), how do we know if some material within the medium has changed (usually lowered) the surface tension? Because of these questions, many investigators simply report the bubble point and the liquid employed. But other complications cloud the meaning of the bubble point as well.

Consider the investigator who measured the bubble point of a 47-mm-diameter disk as described. He then measured the bubble point of a 293-mm-diameter disk of the same medium. The larger housing gathered air from atop the flooded medium into a tube connected to an eyedropper held under water. He increased air pressure on the underside of the medium and looked for the first bubbles out of the eyedropper. He found that the 293-mm-diameter disk had a lower bubble point than the 47-mm-diameter disk. Did this mean the larger disk was not well sealed in the housing? That air leaked around the disk? Or did it mean there were pinholes or other imperfections in the large disk?

Reti (1977) solved the problem. If the operator with the 47-mm-diameter disk had employed a sensitive airflow meter rather than looking for bubbles, he would have found a bubble point closer than he did with the 293-mm-diameter disk. And, of course, looking for the first flow of bubbles from the larger disk rather than measuring the airflow rate leads to errors. Johnston and Meltzer (1980) asked seven different people to say when they saw a steady flow of bubbles from an eyedropper. The responses varied from 5 to 50 mL/min.

4.2   The Extended Bubble-Point Test

ASTM F316 describes the extended bubble-point test but with little discussion. Essentially, after the bubble point is reached, air pressure is continually increased while making note of the fast-increasing airflow rate. But before that, a record is made of airflow through the dry medium vs. pressure. Yet — and this is important — in the second step the medium is soaked with liquid of low vapor pressure. Why? Increasing air pressure must blow liquid out of smaller holes, not evaporate the liquid. Figure 4.2a illustrates the kind of data obtained from two different filter membranes of equal thickness and porosity but differing in averaged pore sizes. The upper, straight lines show airflow velocities emitting from the tops of the dry membranes, U. Membrane B has smaller pores. Recall the slopes of the straight lines in Figure 2.1.

After soaking each membrane with a nonvolatile liquid (such as a silicon oil) and slowly applying air pressure from underneath, a small flow of air begins to emerge from the tops, represented by Line D. That flow results from air dissolving in the liquid then diffusing to the top face where, at lower pressure, it comes out of solution giving the appearance of hydrodynamic

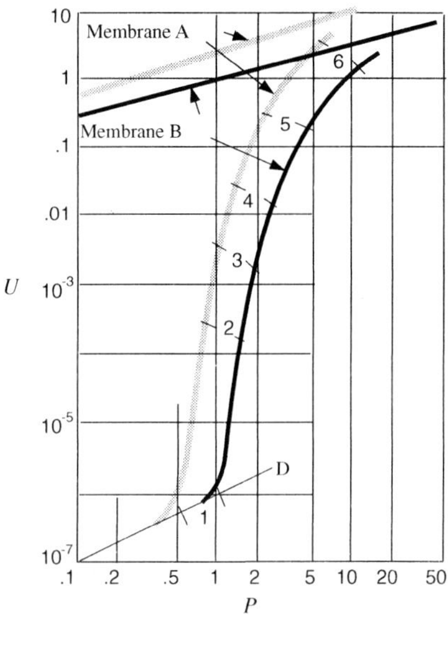

(a)

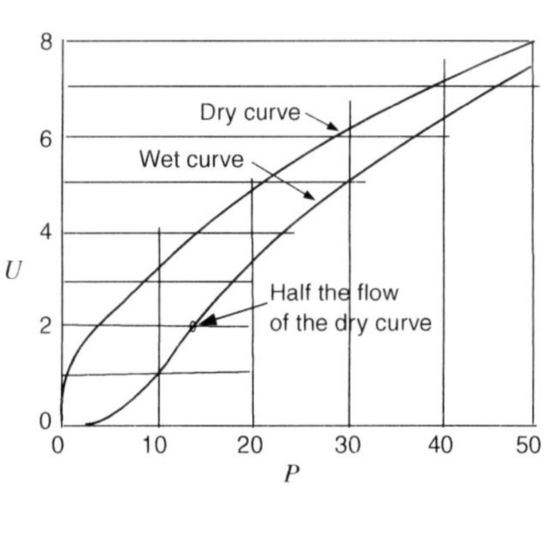

(b)

FIGURE 4.2

(a) Examples of the extended bubble-point test. U = volumetric velocity of gas emitting from the top of a filter membrane at 0 gauge pressure. P = gauge pressure from underneath. Both measurements are in arbitrary units. The upper, straight lines, for two different membranes, show gas flows through dry membrane vs. pressure. The lower, D Line shows diffusion gas flows through the membranes before any pores on the top surface blow open with increasing pressure from underneath. The bubble points are at the two points numbered 1. Other numbered points are discussed in the text as alternative bubble points. (b) Linear/linear plots of the black lines in Figure 4.2 (a).

flow. Line D has a slope of 1.0 because the solubility of air in the liquid is directly proportional to pressure. The vertical location of Line D depends, of course, on the solubility of air in the liquid and on the diffusion rate of the air molecules to the upper side. It also depends on the porosity of the membrane, meaning the volume and thickness of the liquid. Notice that Line D is the same for both membranes when both have the same porosity and thickness; which is to say, Line D is not a function of pore sizes. For detailed calculations around this diffusion rate see Reti (1977) or Treybal (1980).

As gas pressure increases from underneath, to about $P = 0.4$ units in the example of Membrane A (the gray curve), liquid rises to the top and the gas diffusion rate increases because of the shortening columns of liquid. Near $P = 0.5$ gas blows open the largest pores on the upper face of the medium, beginning the fast rise in airflow rate with increasing pressure. Johnston and Meltzer (1980) define the bubble point as Point 1, where the downward extension of the steep curve crosses Line D. And, as mentioned above, the bubble point depends on the position of Line D. Membrane B (the black curve) has a higher bubble point (also labeled Point 1) because of smaller pores. Many investigators, however, lacking sensitive gas flow meters with which to see Line D or relying on the naked eye, do not discern any gas flow until about Points 2, 3, or 4. In each of these two examples Point 3 is 0.001 of the dry-curve lines. That is, Point 3 in either curve corresponds to 0.999 of the pore-size distribution in searching for the largest pores. ASTM F316 prescribes a linear/linear plot of U vs. P. Thus, Figure 4.2b shows such a plot for the black curves in Figure 4.2a. ASTM F316 neither mentions Line D in Figure 4.2a nor addresses the precision of the measurement of the bubble point. Notice the dry curve in Figure 4.2b. As driving pressure falls to zero, the airflow does not, as mentioned in Section 2.3 (when rated pore diameters are smaller than 0.5 µm.)

Many investigators, in presenting such a linear/linear plot, show a straight line for the dry curve emitting from the origin, and they show that the wet curve actually joins the dry curve. They make two errors: their measurements of U and P are in error; and they employ a volatile liquid to soak the medium. If the bubble-point procedure is ever standardized, the report of the bubble point must include the gas flow ratio of wet curve to dry curve to show how far out in the distribution one must reach to find the largest pores. Is it Point 1, Point 2, Point 3, or where? While Reti (1977) did make us aware of Line D in Figure 4.2a, he did not define the bubble point.

Point 6 in Figure 4.2a is half the airflow rate through dry media. Many writers, influenced by ASTM F316, refer to Point 6 as the representing the mean flow pore, when, of course, it corresponds to the middle or median. Moreover, it does not even correspond to the laminar flow middle. The slope of the dry lines (recalling Figure 2.1) tells us that laminar gas flow is diluted with Knudsen flow. Thus, gas flow from the top surface of the medium is not altogether a function of pore diameters to the fourth power. Some of the flow is a function of diameters squared. Moreover, even if the pores are large enough so that Knudsen flow is absent, the flow can be in the inertia range

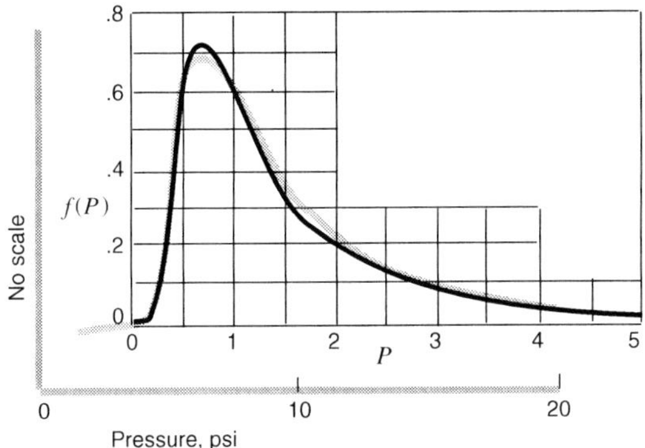

FIGURE 4.3
Differential plots of extended bubble-point data. Gray curve: experimental data reported on page 119 of Meltzer (1987) for a sub-µm-rated membrane (Courtesy of Marcell Dekker). Black curve: plot of Equation 4.1.

when high pressures are necessary to blow open the small pores. So airflow is also a function of pore diameter to less than the fourth power.

For the present example, assume that gas flow out of the top face is a function of pore diameters cubed and relate that to experimental data reported on page 119 of Meltzer (1987), shown as the gray curve in Figure 4.3. That curve is a differential plot of the wet/dry ratio of Figure 4.2a-type data vs. increasing pressure. While the horizontal axis shows pressure values, the vertical axis shows no units. Now compare the gray curve to the black curve. The black curve is described by

$$f(P) = [4.02]\frac{(1/P)^3}{\exp(2/P)} \tag{4.1}$$

Equation 4.1 is a variation of Equation 3.3 in which X, pore size, has been replaced with $1/P$, with P as pressure (recalling Figure 4.1) and the scale factor, β, in Equation 3.3 is arbitrarily set as 2.0. Figure 4.3 shows a direct comparison between experimental results and the theory based on Math Model A in Section 3.2. The experimental work showing the gray curve in Figure 4.3 involved three different airflow meters and pressure gauges of varying sensitivities so as to obtain precise measurements over the wide range of values.

Sampson (2001) reports the results of extended bubble point analyses on 71 different paper handsheets (instead of filter membranes). He reports doing the tests in accordance with ASTM F316. The weights of the paper sheets differed from 20 to 60 g/m². But neither thicknesses nor densities are reported. We assume the heavier sheets have smaller pores. While Sampson does not show the type of data shown in Figure 4.2a, he does report the mean (not middle) pore radii, μ, for each sheet as well as the standard deviation, σ. Interestingly, with decreasing μ, he found increasing σ/μ ratios. Specifically, with μ ranging from 2 to about 36 μm, he found the correlation $\sigma = 0.462\mu + 0.223$. Which is to say, when $\mu = 35$, then $\sigma/\mu = 0.462$, and when $\mu = 2$, then $\sigma/\mu = 0.579$.

That trend can be explained as follows: Smaller pores require higher gas pressures to open. That, in turn, leads to higher gas flows, up into the inertia flow range (Figure 2.1) where flows are no longer a function of pore radii to the fourth power, r^4, but to lower powers. Recall Equation 3.3, where $\alpha = 5$ for viscous flow (r^4). In that case, $\sigma/\mu = \alpha^{-0.5} = 0.447$, and when $\alpha = 4$, nearing inertia flow (r^3), $\sigma/\mu = \alpha^{-0.5} = 0.500$.

Hernandez et al. (1996) analyzed many track-etched membranes by the extended bubble-point test and found, as expected, (with the straight-through sub-μm pores) very narrow pore-size distributions. They also provide a discussion of Kundsen and Poiseuille (laminar) flow.

4.3   The Integrity Test

As Jornitz and Meltzer (2001) explain, the Federal Drug Administration (FDA) mandates that a filter cartridge containing a membrane meant to sterilize a stream must be tested for integrity before filtration proceeds as well as afterwards. In such a test the investigator measures the airflow rate before the bubble point (Line D in Figure 4.2a) then raises the pressure to find the bubble point.

Measuring the airflow rate (or any gas flow rate) in the diffusion zone (Line D in Figure 4.2a,) is referred to as a forward flow test or pressure hold test or flow decay test. The test proceeds as follows. After installing a sterile cartridge into a sterile housing with the exit valve closed (pinching off the line feeding a bottling machine), flood the assembly with the liquid to be filtered while opening an upper vent to exhaust air displaced by the liquid. Assuming the liquid has indeed filled all pores (knowing the liquid does wet the medium), isolate the liquid from the supply line, close the upper vent, then open a second valve on the exit stream. That second exit stream does not feed the bottling machine in case the integrity test fails.

Introduce air on the upstream side at a pressure of about half of the expected bubble point. Notice the flow of liquid being pushed out of the housing. When that flow stops, when all liquid on the upstream side has passed through the membrane, measure the resulting airflow rate through the liquid-filled membrane. Knowing the area of the membrane in place, deduce the velocity of air emitting from the downstream face of the membrane. That velocity must correspond to previous laboratory measurements on such a membrane, as in Line D in Figure 4.2a. If the velocity is as expected, the installed cartridge has integrity. If the air velocity, U, is higher than expected, say by a factor of 10 (consider the examples in Figure 4.2a), go ahead anyway with increasing the pressure to find the bubble point. If the bubble point is no lower than about 0.9 of the expected bubble point, consider the membrane safe to use.

Alternatively, once the liquid volume upstream from the filter media has emptied, close the air feed valve and observe the decline in airflow rate, and thus perform the flow decay test. That rate of decay is a function of the air volume on the upstream side, the area of the membrane, as well as the diffusion rate of air through the liquid in the membrane. Suppliers of membrane filters offer instruments to perform such tests, which can be attached to the filter assembly. Those instruments measure Line D in Figure 4.2a as well as the bubble point. Indeed, such instruments even print out results that can be kept as FDA-required records of such tests.

But what if, in the example of Figure 4.2a, a wet curve starts out at $P = 0.1$. That is, the U scale shows an airflow of 10^{-5} units (instead of 10^{-7}) because of some pinholes or other imperfections in a membrane. In that case, the developing line would have a slope parallel to the dry curve instead of a slope of 1.0 as Line D. Schroeder et al. (1986) addressed that case. They selected 15 cartridges of membrane filters that showed indications of pinhole leaks and deliberately tested those cartridges with microbe-filtration tests. Their table of results shows the expected filtration efficiencies if indeed pinholes let pass some of the test microbes. They reasoned that a certain portion of a feed stream carries unfiltered microbes through the oversize holes. They then compared that list to the filtration efficiencies actually achieved.

Filtration efficiency is expressed as the ratio, R, of the number of microbes in the feed stream to the number in the filtrate. Because R is large, the term $\log R$ is employed. The investigators found that the results of the integrity test implied that the worst case situations would result in $\log R$ values ranging from 5.1 to 5.9. However, the actual filtration test showed $\log R$ values of 6.9 to 7.9. Indeed, with one cartridge, the implied $\log R = 3.5$ turned out to be the actual $\log R = 6.4$.

4.3.1 Calculations around the Flow Decay Test

The permeability, k, of the liquid in the membrane of a given thickness to the diffusive flow of air or other gas is

$$k = \frac{n}{tAP} = \frac{kmol}{s \cdot N} \tag{4.2}$$

where
    n/t = gas-flow rate, kmol/s
    A = membrane area, m^2
    P = gauge pressure on the upstream side, N/m^2 (with 0 gauge pressure on the downstream side)

From the ideal gas law,

$$n = \frac{PV}{RT}$$

where
    V = volume of air space on the upstream side, m^3
    R = gas constant, 8.314 N·m/kmole·K
    T = K = °C + 273

Write the loss in pressure with time as

$$\frac{-P}{t} = \frac{kRTAP}{V} \text{ or } \frac{-d(P_0 - P)}{dt} = \frac{dP}{dt} = \frac{kRTA(P_0 - P)}{V}$$

where
P_0 = gauge pressure at time zero
P = pressure at time t

Rearranging for integration,

$$\frac{kRTA}{V} \int_0^t dt = \int_{P_0}^{P} \frac{dP}{(P_0 - P)}$$

After integration and rearrangement,

$$k = \frac{1}{t} \frac{V}{RTA} \ln\left[\frac{P_0}{P_0 - P}\right] \tag{4.3}$$

In the case where the air volume on the upstream side of the filter medium, V_m, is not known, the instrument contains a space of known volume V_i, from which V_m is deduced using $V_m = V_i P_0 / P$. But we must know the area of the filter medium tested.

4.3.2 Example of a Flow Decay Test

Hofmann (1984) pre-wet a 0.2-μm-rated, pleated membrane cartridge 10 inches long and applied an air pressure of 2700 mbar ($2.7 \cdot 10^5$ N/m²). Then he closed the air supply line. During 180 seconds the pressure fell 18 mbar. From Equation 4.3

$$\ln\left[\frac{P_0}{P_0 - P}\right] = \ln\left[\frac{2700}{2682}\right] = \ln 1.00671 = 6.689 \times 10^{-3}$$

Hofmann (1984) mentions that the volume of upstream air was 0.0013 m³. We assume the area of the membrane was 0.5 m², the temperature was 300 K, and from Equation 4.3, deduce

$$k = \frac{1}{180} \times \frac{1.3 \times 10^{-3}}{8.314 \times 300 \times 0.5} \times 6.689 \times 10^{-3}$$

$$= 3.87 \times 10^{-11} \frac{kmol}{s \cdot N}$$

The initial molecular flow of air was

$$\frac{n}{t} = kAP = 3.87 \times 10^{-11} \times 0.5 \times 2.7 \times 10^5 = 5.26 \times 10^{-6} \ kmol/s$$

Said in another way, the initial velocity of air leaving the downstream face was

$$U = \frac{5.26 \times 10^{-6} kmol}{s} \times \frac{m^3}{22.4 kmol \times 0.5 m^2} = 4.7 \times 10^{-5} m/s$$

4.4 The Drainage Test

The drainage test proceeds as follows. Weigh a sample of the filter medium. Measure the bulk volume. Soak it with any liquid, volatile or not, of known density. Weigh the soaked medium. Deduce the volume of liquid within the medium and thus the porosity of the medium. On the top surface apply a slowly increasing pressure of gas and measure the cumulative volume of liquid draining from the bottom face. But do not apply enough gas pressure on the top face to, in effect, perform an upside-down, bubble-point test. Plot the decrease in liquid saturation as a function of increasing pressure. Figure 4.4 shows the classical kind of plot (Scheidegger 1963; Bear 1972). *J* is called the Leverett function. Bear (1972) further reports that the data plots as an essentially straight line, such as in Figure 4.5, called a Brooks-Corey plot. The slope of a line is a function of the surface tension of the liquid.

Haring and Greenkorn (1970), examining a bed of spheres, suggest that while pore-size distributions follow a gamma distribution (with no further comments), the drainage curve follows the beta distribution, of the specific form

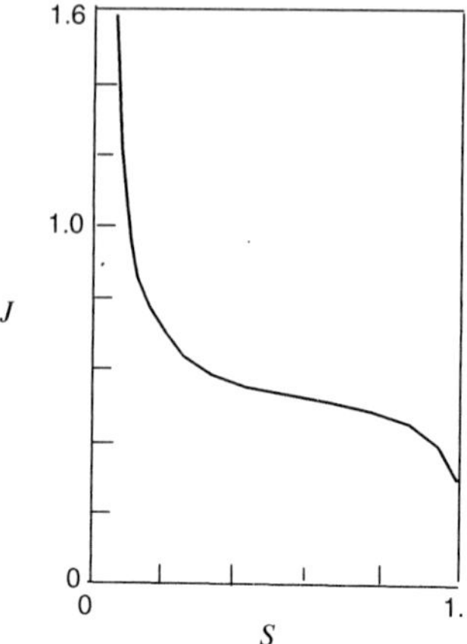

FIGURE 4.4
Plot of drainage data.
    S = saturation

$$J = \frac{P}{\gamma}\left(\frac{B}{\varepsilon}\right)^{1/2}$$

where
    P = pressure, N/m^2
    γ = surface tension of the liquid, N/m
    B = permeability (Equation 1.4), m^2
    ε = porosity

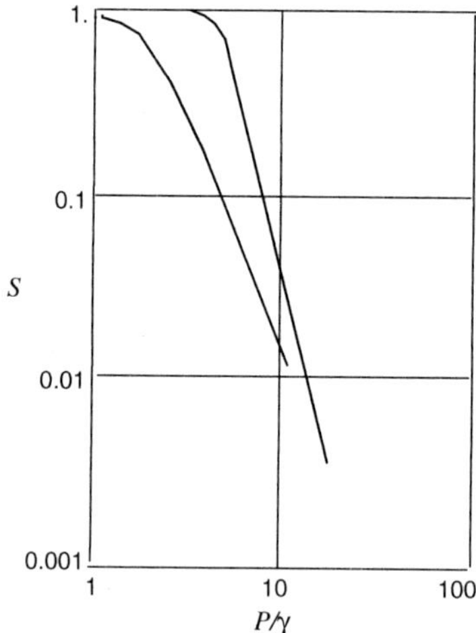

FIGURE 4.5
An alternative plot of drainage data, on log/log paper. S = saturation; P = pressure; and γ = surface tension of the liquid, affecting the slope.

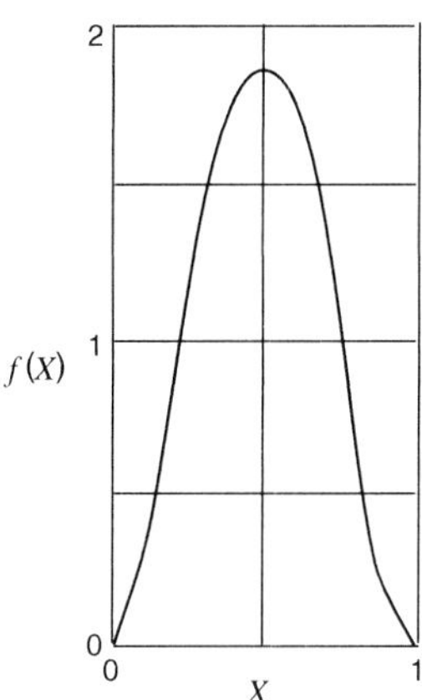

FIGURE 4.6
Plot of Equation 4.4.

$$f(X) = [30]X^2(1-X)^2 \qquad (4.4)$$

where X = pore diameters, from 0 to the maximum of 1.0 unit.

Equation 4.4 is plotted in Figure 4.6. Under that curve 90% of the population lies between X = 0.2 and 0.8, and 80% between 0.25 and 0.75. Haring and Greenkorn (1970) came to Equation 4.4 since a plot of their drainage data followed a Figure 4.4-type of curve. That is, they suggest that the plot is described by an equation of the type

$$f(P) = [3.23]\left(\frac{1}{P}\right)^2\left(1-\frac{1}{P}\right)^2 \qquad (4.5)$$

That is, X, pore diameter, in Equation 4.4 can be expressed as pressure, P, via $1/P$. To understand what Haring and Greenkorn are saying, consider the following. A plot of Equation 4.5, that is, $f(P)$ vs. P, from P = 1 to P =14, shows a curve peaking at $f(P)$ = 0.20 for P = 2.0. At that point, P = 2.0, the cumulative area under the curve (from P = 1.) is 0.13. Which is to say that in a drainage test, 0.13 of the liquid has been expelled so that the saturation has fallen to 1 − 0.13 = 0.87. See in Figure 4.7 that at P = 2.0, saturation, S, is 0.87. Then, at P = 14, in Equation 4.5, the cumulative area of the curve rises to 0.862, meaning the saturation has fallen to 1 − 0.86 = 0.14. See in Figure 4.7 that at P = 14, then S = 0.14. Notice that the shape of the curve in Figure 4.7 resembles that of Figure 4.4.

Miller and Tyomkin (1986), employing drainage tests on microporous membranes, report the narrow kind of distributions shown in Figure 3.4 and Figure 4.6. That is, the largest pore is about three times the size of the smallest pore. Apparently the average pore size deduced by the drainage

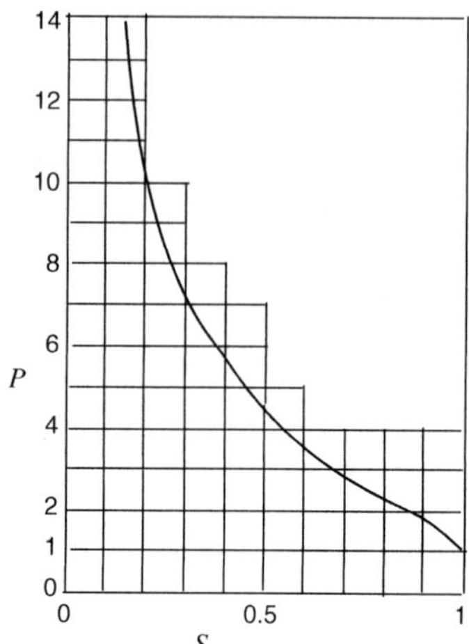

FIGURE 4.7
A roundabout plot of Equation 4.5. *S*, saturation, corresponds to 1.0 minus the cumulative area under curve 4.5.

test corresponds to the flow-averaged pore size deduced by liquid permeability using Equation 1.8.

4.5   The Mercury-Intrusion Test

The mercury-intrusion test begins with placing a porous material in a chamber and pulling out the air, then pushing in mercury with increasing pressure while keeping track of the increased volume of mercury entering as a function of the driving pressure. Mercury approaches all faces of the porous material, not just one face. When it is apparent that the pores are filled, the pressure is slowly reduced. Since mercury does not wet the pore walls (the opposite of Figure 4.1), it wants to get out. The volume coming out is tracked as a function of declining pressure.

With microporous plastic membranes, the pressure needed to fill the pores is likely to compress the membrane, in which case the results have no meaning. But in the case of rigid materials, such as sintered particles of glass, metal, or minerals, the results have some meaning. Conner et al. (1984) and Coyne at al. (1986) provide data for the plot in Figure 4.8. Pore radii are proportional to the reciprocal of pressure (see Figure 4.1 caption).

The term hysteresis refers to the two different curves, *in*trusion and *ex*trusion. One explanation for the two separate curves focuses on the likely difference in wetting angles (θ in Figure 4.1): one angle in (actually a

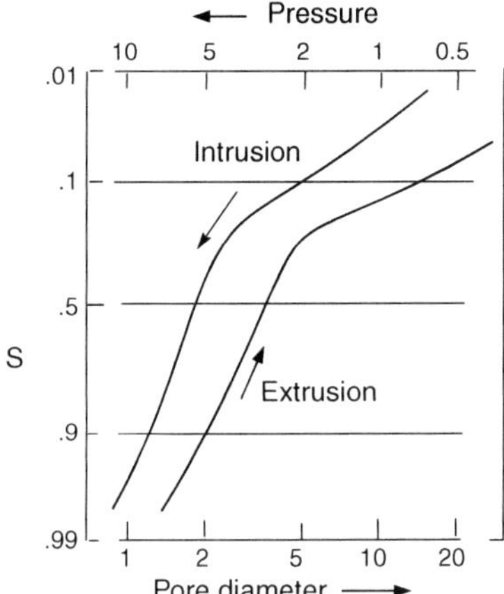

FIGURE 4.8
Curves seen in mercury intrusion studies. S = saturation of the porous medium, probability scale. Pressure: arbitrary units, log scale. Pore diameter: arbitrary units corresponding to 1/pressure. The extrusion curve differs from the intrusion curve.

nonwetting angle) and another angle out. However, Conner et al. (1984) write that the contact angle does not change with the direction of flow for three reasons:

- Mercury does not wet the pore walls, so there can be no consideration of wet-dry history.

- Mercury does not know if it is entering or leaving. The two curves are reproduced when mercury is again forced in and allowed out.

- Intrusion curve occurs as mercury is forced through pore throats, during which time chambers fill. The extrusion curve occurs as chambers empty with mercury passing through throats that are already flooded, thus offering less surface tension forces.

4.6   The Oil-Penetration Test

Like the extended bubble-point test, the oil-penetration test apparently measures the pore-size distribution on the face layer of a filter medium. While the test has been applied to paper sheets, this writer is not aware of it being applied to other filter media. The test proceeds as follows. Lay a sheet onto a pool of black oil. Measure the elapsed time during which the top surface changes from white to darkening shades of gray. The rate of oil penetration for pore radii r, according to Washburn (1921), is

$$\frac{dz}{dt} = \frac{r\gamma \cos\theta}{4\eta z} \tag{4.6}$$

where

dz/dt = instantaneous velocity, distance vs. time, of oil filling a vertical pore of radius r

γ = surface tension of the oil, the force wanting to fill a pore (a tube) acting at the wetting angle, θ. Recall Figure 4.1. Here, assume that $\cos\theta = 1$

η = viscosity of the oil.

Integrating,

$$z^2 = \frac{r\gamma t}{2\eta} \quad \text{or} \quad z = \left[\frac{r\gamma t}{2\eta}\right]^{0.5} \tag{4.7}$$

which is to say that a plot of increasing darkness (comparable to z) vs. the square root of time, provides the indication of the pore-size distribution. Corte and Lloyd (1966) provide linear/linear plots of such data. On plotting their data (two sets, not shown here) on the log/probability paper in Figure 3.1, using the vertical scale as increasing darkness (data from 0.15 to 0.80) and the horizontal scale as seconds$^{0.5}$, on a log scale, the plots follow the slopes in Figure 3.1.

The reader who inspects the papers of Corte and Lloyd (1966) and of Dodson and Sampson (1996) will see that those authors refer to many oil penetration studies done by other people, who do not report their raw data. The other people state that in deducing the mean pore diameters, μ, of paper handsheets, along with the standard deviations, σ, the σ/μ ratios are not constant (not consistent with the gamma distribution). Thus, Corte and Lloyd, then Dodson and Sampson, conclude that the various paper handsheets of the other people differed in the degrees of randomness by which fibers were laid down.

This writer is not aware of any other oil penetration studies. Perhaps the experimental setup has not been fine tuned. That is, what sort of light source and reflective-light measuring device are required? What sort of device is required to lay the sheet onto the pool of oil, at time zero?

5

Particles in Fluids

5.1 Introduction

The point of filtration is to separate particles from a fluid before sterilization. A variety of measurements are employed to judge the clarity of the fluids. Those measurements are used to compare a filtrate to the feed stream as a way of measuring filtration efficiency, which is discussed in Chapter 6. Moreover, some fluids, such as parenteral liquids, must be free of particles or nearly free. This chapter addresses the often misunderstood subject of particle-size distributions in fluids.

We begin by examining the various meanings of clarity. One meaning stresses particle-size distribution: the sizes of individual particles, as well as the numbers or masses of each size of each size range. Because different writers measure and express both particle size and size distribution in different ways, it is important for the investigator to understand these differences.

5.2 Clarity of Streams

Clarity means visual appearance. To assign numbers to appearance, a turbidity scale is used. A fluid is clear when its turbidity is below a certain reading. When filtration is employed to sterilize a liquid, look for live microbes in the filtrate. Store a sample of the filtrate at a warm temperature for a few days and see if it becomes cloudy or gives off a gas. Or place a sample in a petri dish and later count the numbers of colonies, each colony corresponding to one original microbe. One definition of sterility is less than one live microbe per 100 mL. One definition of clarity is no more than five particles per liter larger than a diameter of 25 μm and not more than 50 particles larger than 10 μm. Particle counts are determined with commercially available, automatic particle counters.

To determine the mass concentration of solids in a liquid, pass a sample of the liquid through some very fine filter paper or membrane and weigh the recovered solids. Some writers call this measurement the gravimetric level of the particles. In some cases the recovered particles are so few and so small that a judgment of the particle concentration lies only in the degree to which the filter has been stained, if indeed the particles have a different color than the paper or the membrane.

When water that appears to be clear is fed to a reverse osmosis unit, the clarity of that water is measured by passing a sample through a standard-grade microporous membrane to see how much water can be filtered before the membrane plugs up with accumulated solids. That measurement is the silt density index described in Section 13.3.5. Clarity can denote the concentration of oil dispersed in water, or vice versa. Clarity can have other special meanings. For example, in the paint industry or where a creamy or opaque lotion is the product, the liquid must be free of globs but contain small particles. Thus, clarity, in this case, means a small number of globs, where small is defined. When a liquid is proclaimed free of fibers, the analyst must report the size of the smallest fibers (in both length and diameter) he or she is able to observe.

We can examine the particle-size distribution in a fluid. But, before doing that, we must address the meaning of size. If we are to write a standard method of reporting particle-size distributions, we must first agree on the procedure for measuring and reporting sizes. Indeed, as will be seen in Chapter 6, when we compare particle-size distribution in the feed stream to that in the filtrate, to reach a measure of filtration efficiency, we must agree on how we are going to make that comparison. The two sections that follow discuss methods of measuring particle sizes and the different meanings of particle-size distributions.

5.3 The Meanings of Particle Size and How to Measure It

When a particle is spherical, the meaning of size, diameter, or volume is straightforward. And if we know the density of particles we can deduce their mass. If a particle is a well defined crystal, we can possibly agree on what we mean by size, even if the particle has some irregular shape. Furthermore, using one of many kinds of commercially available automatic particle counters, we can take a statistically significant number of counts by size and thus reach a meaningful particle-size distribution.

Size can mean the longest end-to-end distance seen under a microscope when viewing the particle lying heavy side down. Indeed, an instrument called an image analyzer projects a microscopic view of particles collected on a filter surface onto a TV-like screen and scans it, counting particles of a given size. By viewing many portions of the area of the filter surface, enough counts are obtained to reach a statistically significant number.

Size can mean volume. One type of automatic particle counter, the electrical-resistance type, counts particles suspended in an electrolyte by drawing the suspended solids through an orifice with electrodes on either side of it. As a single particle moves through the orifice, the instrument senses an increase in resistance between the electrodes. The greater the resistance, the larger the volume of the particle. Obviously, the concentration of particles must be low enough so that two or more particles do not pass through at once. When they do, the instrument counts one large particle rather than two or more small ones and thus commits an error called coincidence.

Size can mean the area of a shadow cast by a particle as it passes under a light. An instrument called an optical counter senses particles as they flow by suspended in either a liquid or a gas. The less light passing from the emitter to the receiver, the larger the particle. And like the electrical resistance counter and, indeed, the image analyzer, the optical counter can commit errors of coincidence.

In most fluids with broad ranges of particle sizes, the numbers of small particles are orders of magnitude greater than the numbers of large particles (as seen in Section 5.4). To avoid coincidence with the small particles, present dilute concentrations to the particle counter. To obtain a good count of large particles, examine three or more samples of the liquid, while not considering the counts of small particles where coincidence occurs. Like the meaning of the largest pore on the face of a filter as determined by the bubble point method in Section 4.1, the meaning of the largest particle is statistical. Similarly, the meaning of the smallest particle is a function of the sensitivity with which the counter can discern small particles; there is a limit to what small sizes counters can see. All three of the described automatic particle counters are calibrated with spherical particles of either glass or latex beads. Such spheres are available in separate batches where in each batch all spheres are essentially the same size and many different sizes are available in separate batches.

5.4   Particle-Size Distributions

When counting different-sized particles, the instruments described sort particles into narrow size ranges. For example, the electrical resistance counter sorts volume measurements into ranges within each of which the volume of the largest particle is twice that of the smallest. That is, in each range the largest particle is $2^{1/3}$ or 1.26 times the diameter of the smallest particle. The present discussion follows that procedure in viewing the number of particles in each size range.

A fourth type of instrument directly measures particle mass distribution by sedimentation analysis. For example, when measuring a powder or a dust, a well stirred suspension is placed in an x-ray beam. The particles begin to settle. The larger particles settle faster than the smaller ones. The instrument provides a continuous line and cumulative mass printout of the mass distribution on a scale from 0 to 1.0 (0 to 100%) vs. the Stokes diameter. From the data provided by all of the counters described, we can also draw a chart showing the cumulative mass or number vs. particle diameter.

5.5   Comparing Different Particle Counters

In an attempt to reach a standard meaning of particle diameter, the American Society of Testing and Materials (ASTM) gave different laboratories with different types of particle counters a sample of a specific lot of air cleaner (AC) fine grade test dust (essentially silica, also called Arizona road dust). The laboratories were also given standard sized latex beads for calibrating their instruments. Each laboratory was asked to report the cumulative number distribution versus particle diameter for a specific mass concentration. The results of that venture are shown in Figure 5.1 (Johnston and Swanson 1982b). For the most part, all the labs found the same kind of distribution. That is, each of their curves could be superimposed on the others. The only disagreement, aside from the counts of small particles (discussed in Section 5.6.3), was over the meaning of particle diameter.

At the time, the National Fluid Power Association (NFPA) defined diameter as the longest end-to-end distance. Thus, it became obvious that an investigator using a counter other than the image analyzer could simply multiply his or her diameter values by a certain factor to arrive at the NFPA standard meaning of diameter. ASTM F660 teaches the use of Figure 5.1-type data to suggest a standard meaning of diameter for whatever shape particles are being measured. In any event, the investigator reporting a particle-size distribution must report the kind of instruments used and how they were calibrated.

5.6   The Meaning of Particle-Size Distribution in Fine Grade Test Dust

AC fine grade test dust continues to be used in laboratory filtration tests to characterize filter media according to procedures of the ASTM, NFPA, and the Society of Automotive Engineers (SAE). In Figure 5.1, notice that investigators using optical counters reported fewer small particles than did those

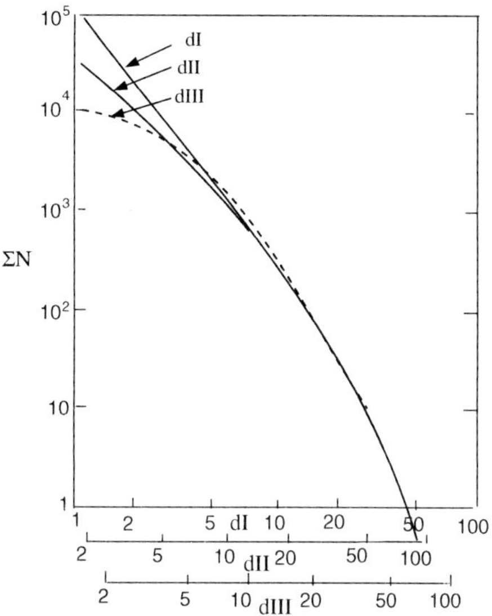

FIGURE 5.1

The particle-size distribution in fine grade test dust according to three different particle counters. ΣN = cumulative numbers of particles per units mass of dust; d = particle diameters, μm; dI = use of electrical resistance counters previously calibrated with spherical beads; dII = use of an image analyzer, where diameter is the longest end-to-end distance; dIII = use of optical counters where the investigators did not calibrate their instruments with spherical beads, as requested in a round robin test, but instead, it was later learned, calibrated their instruments with the dust itself, following the straight line in Figure 5.5. (From Johnston and Swanson 1982b).

using electrical resistance counters. At the time of that study, the workers using the optical counter had prejudged the count of small particles and, we later learned, imposed that view onto their report.

Indeed, the NFPA taught investigators using an optical counter to calibrate their instruments with fine grade test dust, specifying that the distribution was that described by Curve dIII of Figure 5.1. Section 5.6.1 through Section 5.6.5 discusses how the NFPA fell into that error, and how they could have avoided it. This exercise in hindsight enriches an understanding of particle-size distributions.

5.6.1 Deducing Number Distribution from Mass Distribution

In the days before automatic particle counters, the investigator's knowledge of the particle-size distribution in AC fine grade test dust was based solely on the brief data in Table 5.1 provided by the supplier showing a differential mass distribution of particle sizes. Using the data in Table 5.1, we will construct a cumulative number distribution so that we may compare it to the distributions in Figure 5.1. First we construct the graph of Figure 5.2 to

TABLE 5.1

Particle-Size Distribution in AC Fine Grade Test Dust

Stokes diameter, μm	Mass fraction,%
0–5	39 ± 2
5–10	18 ± 3
10–20	16 ± 3
20–40	18 ± 3
40–80	9 ± 3

Note: The original supplier of this material, the AC Spark Plug
Division of General Motors, no longer offers this ma-
terial. It is now offered in various grades by Powder
Technology Inc., Burnsville, Minnesota, and is called
SAE Test Dust, obtained from an Arizona desert.

show the cumulative mass of particles versus diameter. Having drawn the
best estimate of the curve in Figure 5.2, we transfer it to log normal graph
paper in Figure 5.3. Because the curve in Figure 5.3 is a straight line below
a particle diameter of 35 μm, we see a truncated log normal distribution.
Given these data, we will proceed step by step to construct a differential log
normal distribution, showing it as the bottom stair-step dome shaped curve
of Figure 5.4. That is, this bottom series of steps shows the relative masses
(volumes) of particles within the many ranges of particle diameters. To draw
the top stair-step curve of Figure 5.4, representing the relative numbers of
particles in each diameter range, we construct the height of each step from
the bottom curve using the ratio of the height of the bottom step to the
diameter cubed. Finally, we construct the continuous, top (solid-line) curve

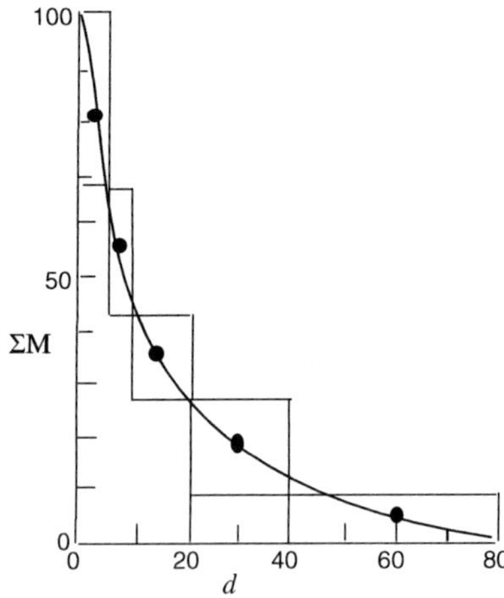

FIGURE 5.2

The particle-size distribution in fine grade test dust deduced from the data of Table 5.1. ΣM =
cumulative mass of particles; d = stokes diameter, μm.

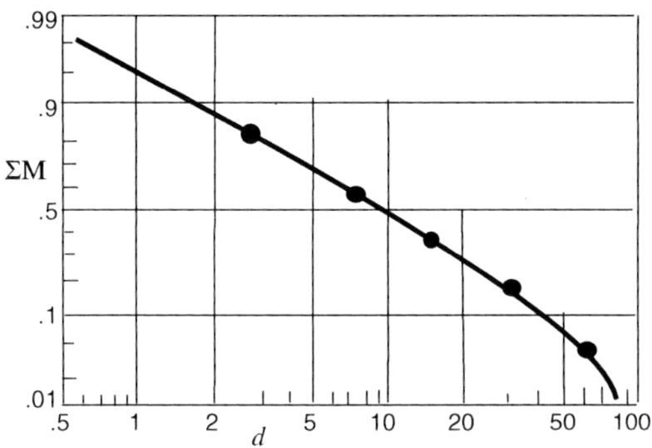

FIGURE 5.3

The points in Figure 5.2 plotted on log/probability paper.

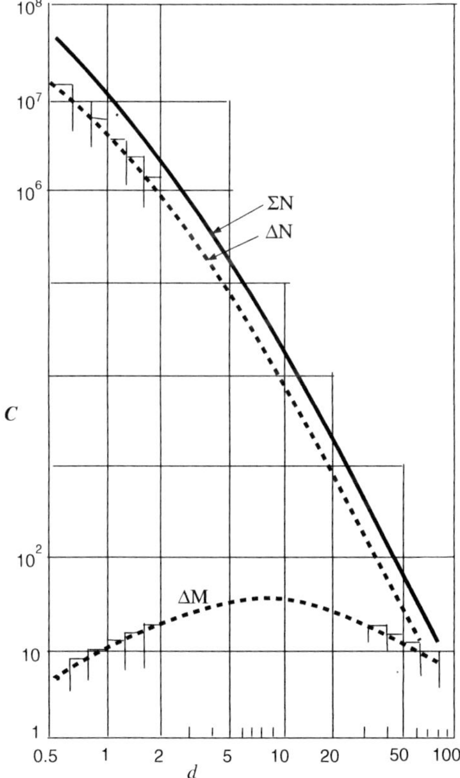

FIGURE 5.4

Other expressions of the data in Figure 5.2. C = relative concentrations of particle diameters, d, μm; ΔM = masses of particles within separate diameter ranges; ΔN = numbers of particles within separate diameter ranges; and ΣN = cumulative numbers of particles, corresponding to Curve dI in Figure 5.1.

of Figure 5.4 by accumulating the stair-step values. The continuous curve represents the cumulative number distribution of particle diameters that we compare to the curves in Figure 5.1. We see more small particles in this curve than are indicated by Curve dIII in Figure 5.1.

5.6.2 Cole's Method of Reaching Number Distribution

We do not know if the late Fred Cole went through the exercise just described, but we know that he painstakingly examined fine grade test dust under a microscope by counting the cumulative numbers of particles in the diameter (longest end-to-end distance) range of 40 to 10 μm (Cole 1966). He then reasoned that the distribution probably follows a log normal distribution, which led him to present an interesting plot of particle counts. The kind of graph paper Cole used is shown in Figure 5.5. When he plotted his cumulative counts of particles vs. the square of the logarithm of the particle diameter in his diameter range of 10 to 40 μm, he obtained a straight line.

5.6.3 An NFPA Standard

Cole's fellow members of the NFPA committee took his plot and ran with it. They extended the straight line as shown in Figure 5.5. From that line

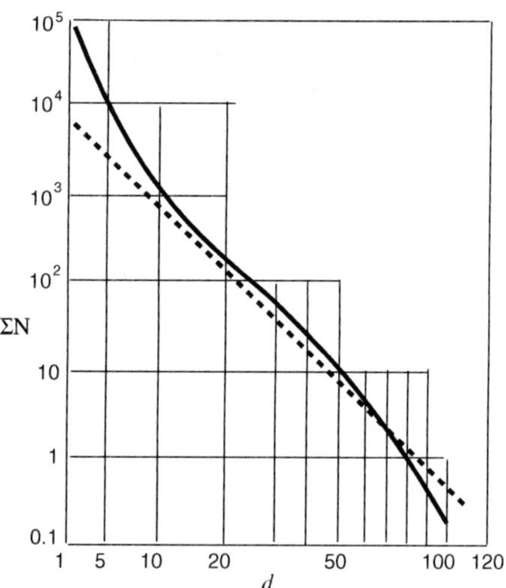

FIGURE 5.5

Another plot of the particle-size distribution in fine-grade test dust. ΣN = cumulative numbers of particles per unit mass of diameters d, μm. The straight line corresponds to Curve dIII in Figure 5.1; the curve, to Curve dI in Figure 5.1. The diameter scale is laid out as $(\log d)^2$. That is, 0 corresponds to $d = 1$, 1 to $d = 10$, and 4 to $d = 100$, following Cole (1966).

they produced a table showing the cumulative counts of particles in a unit mass of fine grade test dust vs. particle diameter in the diameter range of 1 to 100 μm (Fitch 1970). That table became the standard definition of the particle-size distribution in fine grade test dust. Indeed, as mentioned above, operators of optical particle counters were instructed to calibrate their instruments using the data in that table. Thereafter, writers addressing particle-size distributions displayed their data by means of the Figure-5.5 kind of plot with that diameter scale rather than the diameter scale of Figure 5.1. The straight line in Figure 5.5 corresponds to Line dIII in Figure 5.1. That is, the straight line in Figure 5.5 shows fewer small particles and more large particles than are actually present.

By 1974, investigators (Johnston and Schmitz 1974) using the electrical resistance type of counter were displaying particle count data for fine grade test dust using Curve dI in Figure 5.1, instead of dIII, which the NFPA had proclaimed standard. Soon after, Johnston (1978) argued that if an operator twists the dials on an optical counter so that the instrument reads the particle-size distribution as dIII, he or she will obtain incorrect filtration test results. That is, by comparing the particle-size distribution in the filtrate with that of the feed stream, the investigator will obtain misleading data concerning the efficiency with which a filter stops 1-to-10-μm-diameter particles. By 1981, the NFPA realized its error (Campbell and Iwanaga 1981) and instructed investigators to calibrate optical counters with latex beads.

Apparently, the NFPA has not addressed the data in Figure 5.1, which shows that one instrument will report a particle size different from another instrument when both have been calibrated with latex beads. Yet, NFPA tests only employ optical counters. Thus, while an earlier, standard definition of particle size for AC fine grade test dust was the longest end-to-end distance, we see no present attempts to reach a standard definition, except for that taught in 1983 by ASTM F660, which simply suggests comparing the diameter scales in Figure 5.1.

5.6.4 Other Grades of Siliceous Test Dusts

As stated in Table 5.1, the AC Spark Plug Division of General Motors no longer offers Arizona road dust. The new supplier of this siliceous material is Powder Technology, Inc. (PTI). That material is now called SAE Test Dust. PTI offers a description of the particle-size distributions in their products based on an electrical resistance counter analysis (the Coulter Counter™). But rather than describe number distributions, PTI reports normalized, cumulative mass distributions, such as depicted in Figure 5.3, because SAE wants it that way.

Further, in normalizing the data, that is, in expressing it as percentages, PTI assumes that the particle masses (volumes) are zero for particles smaller than diameters of 0.5 μm. That is, on accumulating the mass from the large- to the small-particle end of the spectrum, PTI stops at 0.5 μm, as if all the mass or volume were accounted for.

Having described the three different kinds of particle counters — image analyzer, optical, and electrical resistance — and the sedimentation device, we warn analysts to be cautious using any of these instruments or any kind of instrument for that matter. It is important to understand how an instrument is calibrated, how it measures particle size, and how it computes and reports particle-size distributions. As pointed out above, it is not enough to simply present a single sample to an instrument and push the button.

5.6.5 Analytical Sieves for Deducing Particle-Size Distributions

With relatively large particles at hand, particle-size distribution is deduced by passing particles through various woven-wire screens like the Tyler or U.S. Standard Series. Those screens are available with square openings varying from 38 μm on a side to 1000 μm. Nineteen different screens are available in which the opening on a each is 1.19 times the next smaller one. With the largest screen on top, particles are fed either as dry material or in a slurry, after which the mass of particles retained on each screen is measured. Brittain (2002) discusses this procedure in analyzing pharmaceutical powders.

5.7 Mathematical Models of Particle-Size Distributions

The particle-size distribution in any powder or suspension depends, of course, on the origin of the solids and on whether they have been classified by some method of screening, filtration, or sedimentation. Various mathematical models have been proposed for describing particle-size distributions, Johnston (1976), seeing the particle-size distribution depicted by Curve dI in Figure 5.1, suggests this expression.

$$\Sigma N = A(L - X)X^{-c} \tag{5.1}$$

where
  ΣN = the cumulative numbers of particles per unit volume of a suspension or per unit mass of powder
  A = a concentration index
  L = diameter of the largest particle (Curve dI of Figure 5.1 falls toward zero at some large diameter)
  X = particle diameters
  $-c$ = the (negative) slope on the log/log plot of the straight line where X values are small

Bader (1970) suggests

$$\Sigma N = K(V^{-n} - L^{-n})$$ (5.2)

where
ΣN = cumulative numbers of particles
K = concentration index
V = volume of the particle size of interest
$-n$ = negative slope on the log/log plot of the straight line for small V values
L = volume of the perceived largest particle

Bader (1970) also suggests this expression for the cumulative volumes of particles, V

$$\Sigma V = \frac{nK}{n-1}(V^{1-n} - L^{1-n})$$ (5.3)

where K, n, and L are the same as in Equation 5.2.

In those cases where the volume distribution is expressed as a percentage — that is, we know the sizes of the largest and smallest particles and we have accounted for all those sizes so that we can construct a plot like Figure 5.3 — we can sometimes see this Rosin-Rammler expression as descriptive of that distribution.

$$\Sigma W = \exp-\left(\frac{X}{X_r}\right)^k$$ (5.4)

where
ΣW = cumulative mass fraction, accumulating from high to low diameters
X = particle diameter
X_r = reference diameter
k = a factor addressing the breadth of the distribution

By reference diameter we mean that when the ratio $X/X_r = 1.0$, the value of ΣW is 0.368. Values of k less than 1.0 describe broad distributions; greater than 1.0, narrow distributions. For example, in gas filtration tests, some test aerosols are employed where the geometric standard deviation of the mass distribution is as small as 1.3. Such a narrow distribution can be approximated with $k = 4$ (Johnston 1995).

Obviously, we cannot express a cumulative number distribution as a percentage because we cannot account for the many particles that are too small for a particle counter to see. Recall Figure 5.4. Thus, we cannot report a number-averaged particle size, as some writers have done. But we can report a volume-averaged or mass averaged particle size. In any event, when comparing the particle-size distribution of the feed stream to that of the filtrate, we must not force either distribution to fit a mathematical curve. We will say more on that subject in the next chapter.

Seeing in Figure in 5.3 that the cumulative volume particle-diameter distribution closely approximates a log-normal distribution, Johnston (2000), employing the equation for a log-normal distribution, converted PTI's fine- and medium-grade materials (from their Figure 5.3-type data.) into cumulative-number distributions. The results of the fine grade material matched, as expected, Curve dI in Figure 5.1. Interestingly, the medium-grade material results matched the cumulative-number distribution deduced by the National Institute of Science and Technology (NIST) using image analyses. NFPA now teaches the use of medium grade test dust in filtration tests, instead of the older fine grade test dust. Indeed, NIST offers that test dust suspended in a hydraulic fluid with a certified particle-size distribution so that the investigator can calibrate his optical counter (Eleftherakis and Khalil 1998).

As stated previously, clarity is sometimes defined in terms of the number distribution of particle sizes. In the pharmaceutical industry the standard for large-volume parenteral (injection) liquids specifies less than 5 25-μm-diameter particles per milliliter and less than 10 50-μm particles, as seen in a Figure 5.1-kind of plot (Jornitz and Meltzer 2001).

6

Describing Filtration Efficiency

6.1 Problems of Definition

When I use a word, it means just what *I* choose it to mean — neither more nor less.

(Humpty Dumpty to Alice)
Lewis Carroll's *Through the Looking Glass*

The literature of filtration is somewhat confused; the source of much of the confusion is the variety of ways investigators define and describe filtration efficiency. Chemical engineers refer to filtration as a separation process: particles are separated from a fluid or vice versa. Hence, the efficiency of a given separation process is called filtration efficiency. Many writers speak of the particle removal characteristics of a filter medium. Some, realizing that characteristics do not really say anything, speak simply of removal. Obviously, their eyes are on the fluid rather than on the solids. Other writers, perhaps with eyes on the solids, speak of fluid removal, or particle recovery. In gas filtration, writers refer to arrestance; the filter medium incarcerates the particles.

Many writers sidestep the word efficiency, sometimes for good reason. For example, the term filtration ratio is useful when employing two mathematical rules of thumb in filtration (Section 6.3). Yet many writers confuse filtration ratio with Beta ratio. Other terms used are purification coefficient, decontamination factor, titer reduction ratio, microbiological safety index, retention, rejection, and sieving coefficient.

Each writer coins his or her own word, and it gets worse. Too often we see writing like this: "Penetration is that percentage of the feed particles penetrating the filter medium," using a word in its own definition. Does penetrating mean passing through or going somewhat into the depth of the medium? Does percentage mean the fraction of the mass of particles or the number of particles? Or does it mean some kind of ratio? To describe filtration efficiency, we obviously must compare the clarity or cloudiness of the feed stream to the filtrate. Yet, as discussed in Section 5.2, clarity has different meanings, depending on how we measure it.

When measuring the mass concentration of all particles in the feed stream, C_1, and in the filtrate, C_2, filtration, efficiency, E, is defined as

$$E = (C_1 - C_2)/C_1 \tag{6.1}$$

For example, if the feed stream contains a mass concentration of 100 units per volume, and 12 pass through, then filtration efficiency, E, is 0.88. Many writers prefer to say 88% for the love of percentages. Yet, it is mathematically convenient to employ the term filtration ratio, R.

$$R = C_1/C_2 \tag{6.2}$$

Continuing with the above example where $E = 0.88$,

$$R = 100/12 = 8.33$$

When values of R are very large, as when separating microbes from a feed stream, it is convenient to speak of log R sometimes called the log reduction ratio. For example, when $E = 0.999999$, and $R = 10^6$, then log $R = 6$. During the course of a filtration run, changes occur in filtration efficiency for a variety of reasons. Furthermore, changing the conditions of the operation — for example, changing the velocity or temperature of the fluid — changes filtration efficiency.

Thus, whenever investigators report filtration efficiency, they owe it to their readers to report exactly how they measured efficiency, and, perhaps, why they used that method. They should also report the conditions of the run along with the times in the run when they made measurements.

6.2   When Clarity Means Particle-Size Distributions

Chapter 5 points out the lack of a standard meaning of particle diameter. As shown in Figure 5.1, three different kinds of particle counters, each calibrated with the same size latex beads, report different diameters for a standard test dust. Yet, as Verdegan et al. (1992) have reported, even different kinds of optical counters report different results.

Furthermore, latex beads do not stand up to oil: when we try to use them in oil to calibrate an optical counter that will analyze oil streams. Hence, one solution for oil filtration tests is to use a standard test dust suspended in oil, as mentioned in Section 5.6.3. McBroom (1993) reported the beginning of that remedy. In any event, investigators should explain exactly how they measured particle size. Some writers even fail to tell us if size means radius or diameter. Furthermore, investigators should report their measurements of particle-size distributions, as in Figure 5.4, and not report normalized distributions, as in Figure 5.3, for three reasons:

- In normalizing the data, the investigator assumes knowledge of the distribution of all particle sizes, when in truth he or she is uncertain of the concentration of particles at both ends of the spectrum.

- The reader may want to replicate the work, and one method of checking can be to look at the particle-size distribution in the feed stream, as shown in Figure 5.4.

- When an investigator describes the capacity of a filter medium — the mass of particles fed before the medium plugs, a topic addressed later — the reader is entitled to know the particle-size distribution in the feed stream. Different particle-size distributions in the feed stream lead to different values for the capacity of a medium.

When Alice asked Humpty Dumpty how he can make words mean so many different things, he answered that verbs are stubborn, but he can do anything with adjectives. When his words come around on Saturday night to get their wages he always pays the adjectives extra. ASTM (1986) discourages the conversion of the adjective particulate into a plural noun particulates. ASTM discourages the use of contaminant to mean particle. Call a spade a spade; some contaminants are soluble. But the National Fluid Power Association (NFPA) has continued since 1973 or before to use contaminant, when referring to a specific test dust (NFPA 1990). The Society of Automotive Engineers (SAE) is more precise, referring to that same test dust as particulate contaminant (SAE 1988). Does throughput mean flow rate or volume filtered? People in cross-flow filtration employ their own shop talk, as we discuss in Chapter 12.

6.3 Comparing the Particle-Size Distribution in the Feed Stream to That in the Filtrate

During the course of a filtration test run, investigators routinely measure the clarity of the filtrate and compare it to the clarity or cloudiness of the feed stream. What follows is an example of one such sample comparison, showing two different ways investigators compare particle-size distributions. In Figure 6.1 the ΣN curves (feed and filtrate) represent examples of the cumulative numbers of particles (per unit volume of fluid) vs. particle diameters for a specific time in a filtration run. The ΔN curves show the numbers of particles of individual diameters in the two streams.

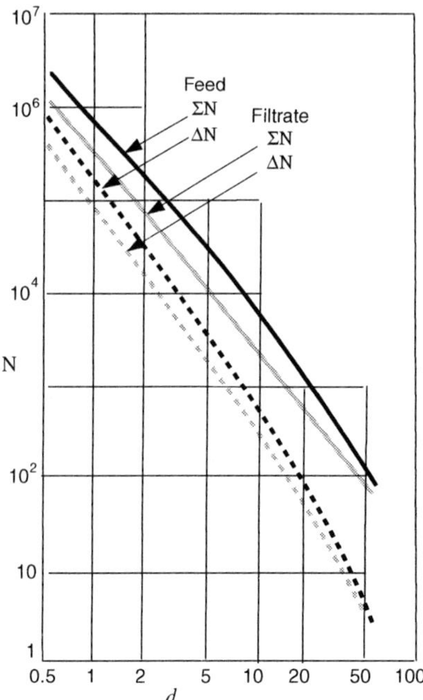

FIGURE 6.1

Examples of particle-size distributions in a feed stream and a filtrate; d = particle diameter, μm; N = numbers of particles per unit volume of liquid; ΣN = cumulative numbers; ΔN = numbers of individual-diameter particles.

From the data in Figure 6.1, Figure 6.2 shows, in the lower line, the efficiencies, E, with which individual-diameter particles, d, were captured by the filter medium. This kind of plot, taught by ASTM F795 and ASTM F796, is made on log/log paper. The right-hand vertical scale shows log R values on a log scale. For example, looking at the lower line, if 100 particles of diameter 5.0 μm are fed to the filter medium and 31 pass through, for a collection efficiency, E, of 0.69, the R value is $100/31 = 3.22$, and log $R = 0.509$.

On the other hand, the NFPA, apparently the first group to try to write a standard filtration test, taught and still teaches that the results should be described by the upper curve in Figure 6.2, although the NFPA does not teach this sort of plot. For example, the upper line in Figure 6.2 shows the filtration efficiency of the numbers of 5-μm and larger particles were stopped with an efficiency of 0.80, for a log R value of 0.699. Some writers have compared the cumulative masses of particles to draw an even higher curve in Figure 6.2.

However, the NFPA does not use the term filtration ratio. Instead, they use the term Beta ratio (with no relationship to the mathematical beta distribution, mentioned in Section 4.4.) Furthermore, the Beta ratio was originally restricted to situations in which the feed stream contained fine grade

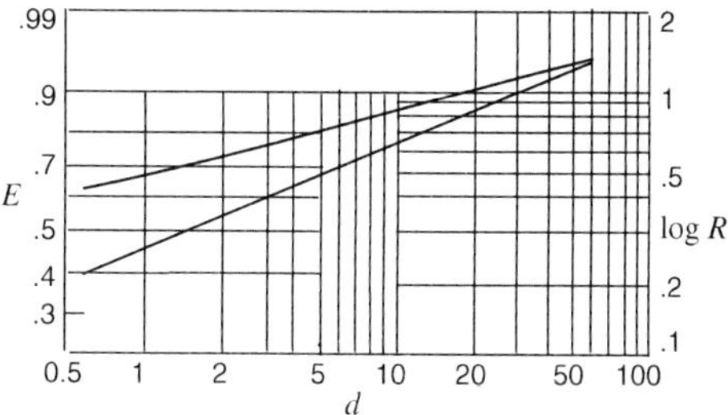

FIGURE 6.2

Plots of data from Figure 6.1 of log R, and filtration efficiency, E, vs. particle diameter, d, μm. The lower line shows the efficiencies with which individual-size particles were captured by the filter medium, in comparing the ΔN curves in Figure 6.1. The upper curve shows the efficiencies with which the numbers of d-diameter and larger particles were captured, in comparing the ΣN curves, that is, in employing Beta-type ratios. Obviously, the upper curve shows higher results. As mentioned in the text, the position and shape of the upper curve is a function of the particle-size distribution in the feed stream, whereas the lower line is not.

test dust. When the feed stream contained coarse grade dust, the NFPA taught the use of the Alpha ratio because such ratios depend on the particle-size distribution in the feed stream. Yet where NFPA has carried their teachings into ISO 16889 and now employs medium grade test dust, instead of fine grade, they still refer to Beta ratios. D'Andrea (2003) shows a table where such Beta ratios are converted to filtration efficiency!

Campbell and Iwanaga (1981) point out that changing the particle-size distribution in the feed stream does indeed change the Beta ratio. They go on to provide a monograph explaining how to convert a Beta ratio obtained from a nonstandard particle-size distribution in the feed steam to the Beta ratio that would have been obtained if fine grade test dust had been used, assuming that the particle-size distribution in the fine grade is that described by Curve dIII of Figure 5.1. In Figure 6.1 the $\Delta N/\Delta N$ ratios in the feed/filtrate, the R values, are independent of the particle-size distribution in the feed stream and are smaller than Beta or Alpha ratios. Many writers do not understand the differences between the $\Delta N/\Delta N$ ratios — the R values — and the $\Sigma N/\Sigma N$ ratios — the Beta-type values. Moreover, as we will discuss later, some writers who compare the numbers of single-size microbes in a feed stream to those in the filtrate employ the Beta ratio.

The investigator who would seek the filtration ratio, R, of, say, only 5-μm particles, with only knowledge of the ΣN curves in Figure 6.1, proceeds as follows. Determine the slopes, S, of the ΣN curves at the 5-μm points. Use those slopes in converting the $\Sigma N/\Sigma N$ ratios to $\Delta N/\Delta N$ ratios via Equation 6.3 (ASTM F795 and ASTM F796).

$$\frac{\Delta N_1}{\Delta N_2} = \frac{\Sigma N_1}{\Sigma N_2} \cdot \frac{S_1}{S_2} \qquad (6.3)$$

where subscript 1 refers to the feed stream and subscript 2 to the filtrate.

SAE, like NFPA, uses fine grade test dust and looks at the Beta ratio, instead of $\Delta N/\Delta N$ as defined by ASTM, and converts that ratio directly to filtration efficiency, E, as illustrated in Figure 6.3, but refers to the Beta ratios as R. On the other hand, some writers show linear/linear plots of either E, or R, or Beta vs. particles diameter. But those plots, like the SAE plot in Figure 6.3, fail to show what the lower line in Figure 6.2 shows. That line indicates that the log R values of individual-size particles are described by

$$\log(\log R) = \log a + n \log d \quad \text{or} \quad \log R = ad^n \tag{6.4}$$

where

    a =   a measure of the overall filtration efficiency
    n =   the degree with which different-size particles are separated
    d =   particle diameter

That is, the lower line of Figure 6.2 provides more information than any other kind of plot. Indeed, that line is useful in explaining two rules of thumb (Johnston 1982a):

- Increasing the thickness of the filter medium by a factor of two results in a two-fold increase in the log R values of all particle sizes.

- Two filter media of equal thickness, where the square of the flow-averaged pore diameter in one is half that of the other, show a two-fold increase of all log R values, provided the fluid velocity is the same. As discussed in Chapter 1, in both cases the fluid driving pressure must be increased by a factor of two to maintain the same fluid velocity.

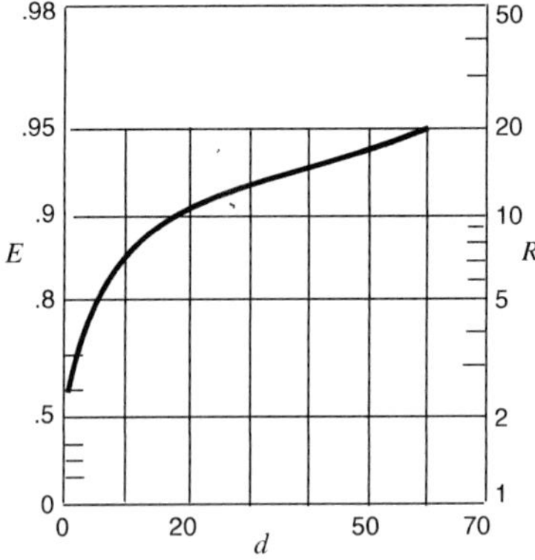

FIGURE 6.3
An SAE method of plotting the upper line in Figure 6.2. Notice that the d scale is linear and the R scale is logarithmic. But here R does not mean the filtration ratios of individual-size particles; it refers to Beta-type ratios.

6.4 Other Comparisons of Clarity

SAE Method J806 and SAE Method J905 look not at particle-size distributions but only at the total mass of particles in the separate streams.

The present writer, using an electric resistance counter to compare particle-size distributions, has seen with SAE test dust in water that the efficiency with which turbidity is filtered corresponds to the efficiency with which 0.5-to-1.0-μm-diameter particles are separated.

6.5 Absolute Filtration

Some suppliers of filter media offer what they call absolute filters (borrowing the name from a famous vodka?). But some absolutes are more absolute than others. Investigators, addressing filtration results with test dusts, suggest that a filtration efficiency greater than 0.98 is absolute. In addressing the capture of microbes, absolute means a filtration efficiency greater than 0.9999999, greater than a log R value of 7, as discussed later.

6.6 Deducing Pore Sizes from Filtration Tests

Do not try to deduce pore sizes from filtration tests. Consider two filter media, each composed of the same material with the same porosity and permeability and thus with the same pore-size distribution but one thicker than the other. In filtration tests, with equal fluid velocities, the thicker medium will be more efficient at stopping all particle sizes. The tests results do not mean that the thicker medium has smaller pores.

Johnston (1975), working with a filter paper, shows how changes in log R values and the filtration efficiencies of given-size particles, E, change with changes in water flow rate, temperature, and kinds of test particles. The data are shown in Figure 6.4.

Any attempt to devise a standard filtration test involves arbitrarily fixing some conditions. Consider the standard test procedure for evaluating filter cartridges designed to clean hydraulic fluids, ISO 16889 (D'Andrea 2003). In real use we expect different results between one test with winter temperatures and another with summer temperatures. However, filter membranes meant to sterilize streams, are rated by pore size, a muddled subject that is discussed Chapter 11.

                                    Fluid Sterilization by Filtration, Third Edition

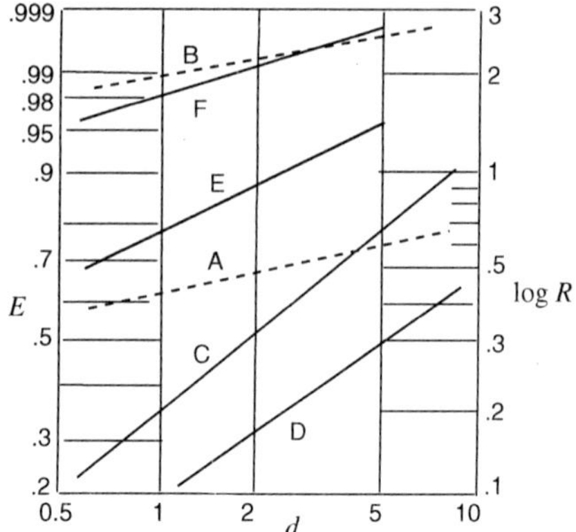

Line	Particle	°F	gal/min•ft^2
A	silica	70	1
B	silica	170	1
C	iron oxide	70	1
D	iron oxide	70	5
E	iron oxide	170	5
F	iron oxide	170	1

FIGURE 6.4

Use of a filter paper to clarify water slurries of silica particles (SAE test dust) or black iron oxide under different conditions. *E* refers to the filtration efficiency of individual-diameter particles d, μm (Johnston 1975).

7

Structure and Permeability of Filter Media

7.1 Random Array Filter Media

This chapter discusses the kinds of filter media most often employed, those composed of random arrays of building materials, such as solvent-cast microporous membranes and sheets or beds of granules or fibers.

7.2 The Kozeny-Carman Constant

As Kozeny, then Carman, devised vocabulary with which to express the viscous permeability of a porous material structure, even Carman (1956) stated that the so-called constant, in the expression now identified by their names, is not really constant. Scheidegger (1963) provides a more recent review. Yet many current writers still treat it as a constant, thus the present review.

The so-called constant, k, is seen in Equation 7.1, relating viscous permeability, B (m^2) in Equation 1.4 and Equation 2.1, to porosity, ε, along with the ratio of the volume of solids, V_s, to the surface area of those solids, A_s.

$$B = \left(\frac{V_s}{A_s}\right)^2 \frac{\varepsilon^3}{(1-\varepsilon)^2 k} \tag{7.1}$$

where k is assumed to be approximately 5.

Equation 7.1 is examined as follows. The volume of the voids, V_o, is related to porosity as

$$\varepsilon = \frac{V_o}{\left(V_o + V_s\right)} \quad \text{so that} \quad V_o = \frac{V_s \varepsilon}{(1-\varepsilon)}$$

Dividing both sides by A_s,

$$\frac{V_o}{A_s} = \frac{V_s}{A_s}\frac{\varepsilon}{(1-\varepsilon)} \tag{7.2}$$

Now, separately, consider an average tube-shaped pore of internal diameter d, and length L, so that the ratio of the internal volume to the internal surface area is

$$\frac{V_o}{A_s} = \frac{\pi\left(d^2/4\right)L}{\pi dL} = \frac{d}{4} \tag{7.3}$$

The hydraulic diameter, by definition, is four times the V_o/A_s ratio, for any shape, such as a square or triangle, and thus is equal to d. Since the surface area of the solids is the same as the surface area of the pores (assuming point contacts of the solids), we can combine Equation 7.2 and Equation 7.3

$$d = \frac{V_s}{A_s}\frac{\varepsilon}{(1-\varepsilon)} \tag{7.4}$$

Suppose the solids are fibers of diameter d_f and length L_f, so that the volume/surface area ratio of an individual fiber is

$$\frac{V_s}{A_s} = \frac{\pi\left(d_f^{\,2}/4\right)L_f}{\pi d_f L_f} = \frac{d_f}{4} \tag{7.5}$$

Or suppose the solids are spheres of diameter d_{sp}

$$\frac{V_s}{A_s} = \frac{\pi(d_{sp})^3}{6\pi(d_{sp})^2} = \frac{d_{sp}}{6} \tag{7.6}$$

From such reasoning, the average pore diameter, d, for either kind of solid is

$$d = \frac{d_f\varepsilon}{(1-\varepsilon)} = \frac{4d_{sp}\varepsilon}{6(1-\varepsilon)} \tag{7.7}$$

Recall from Equation 1.8 that permeability, B, is related to flow-averaged pore diameter, d_F, and is expressed as

$$B = \frac{(d_F)^2 \varepsilon^2}{32} \tag{7.8}$$

In any event, investigators have followed Equation 7.1 with the meanings of V_s/A_s in Equation 7.5 and Equation 7.6.

For fibers, Rushton and Griffiths (1977) consider

$$B = \frac{(d_f)^2}{k} \frac{\varepsilon^3}{(1-\varepsilon)^2} \tag{7.9a}$$

and then proceed to deduce changes in k with changes in ε.

Yet Ergun (1952), for equivalent spheres, considers

$$B = \frac{d_{sp}^{\;2}}{36} \frac{\varepsilon^3}{(1-\varepsilon)^2 k} \tag{7.9b}$$

and reports that k is indeed constant at 4.16.

7.3 The Kozeny Factor for Fibrous Media

For fibrous media Rushton and Griffiths (1977) provide the correlation between ε and k in Equation 7.9a as that in Table 7.1.

TABLE 7.1

Equation 7.9a, k as a Function of ε

ε	0.2	0.3	0.4	0.5	0.6	0.7	0.8	0.9
k	2.7	3.8	4.9	5.8	6.3	6.6	7.2	9.8

Monson (1986), not considering k, calculated the viscous drag of a single fiber held perpendicular to fluid flow and then expanded that to many randomly arrayed fibers packed to a solidity, c. Recall $\varepsilon = 1 - c$. In describing the dimensionless viscous drag, F, as a function of c (verified by actual measurements), he relates these values to permeability, in the notation we use in Equation 1.4, as

$$B = \frac{u\eta z}{\Delta P} = \frac{\pi d_f^{\;2}}{4cF} \tag{7.10}$$

His charts provide the data for Table 7.2.

TABLE 7.2

Equation 7.10, *cF* as a Function of *c* ($c = 1 - \varepsilon$)

c	0.9	0.8	0.7	0.6	0.5	0.4	0.3	0.2	0.1	0.05
cF	25,000	4,400	1,050	330	125	48	16	4.8	1.3	0.38

From Table 7.1 and Table 7.2, Johnston (1989) says that in the range $\varepsilon = 0.1$ to 0.85,

$$\frac{B}{(d_f)^2} = 2.66 \cdot 10^{-3} \left[\frac{\varepsilon(1+\varepsilon)}{(1-\varepsilon)} \right]^2 \tag{7.11}$$

Davies (1973) says that in the range of $c = 0.006$ to 0.3 (ε from 0.7 to 0.994)

$$\frac{B}{(d_f)^2} = \frac{1}{64c^{1.5}\left(1 + 56c^3\right)} \tag{7.12}$$

Equation 7.11 and Equation 7.12 are plotted in Figure 7.1.

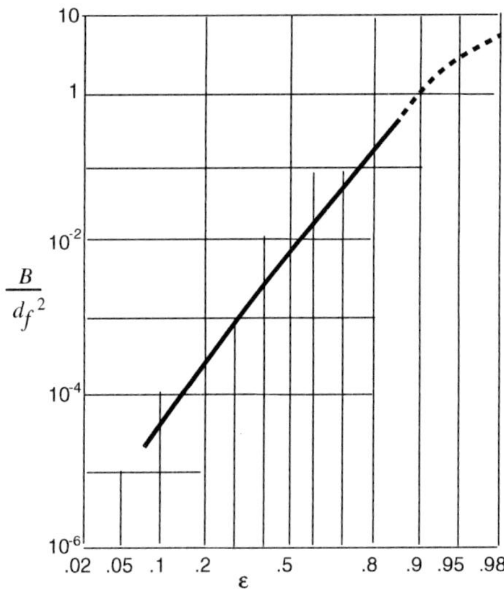

FIGURE 7.1

Permeability, *B*, of fibrous media, with fiber diameters d_f, as a function of porosity, ε. The ε scale is laid out on the probability scale. Equation 7.11 describes the solid curve, Equation 7.12 the broken curve.

7.4 The Kozeny-Carman Factor for Granular Media

When Carman (1937) looked at the permeability of granular beds with porosities, ε, ranging from 0.37 to 0.66, he saw k values ranging from 4.8 to 6.13 but made no attempt to correlate ε with k. And while he suggests that the tortuosity factor, τ, in a bed of spheres is $2^{0.5}$, he does not use that thinking in concluding that on average $k = 5$ (not 5.0). Ergun (1952), often cited, looking at various beds of column packing materials, assuming the volume/surface ratios are those of equivalent spheres, concludes that $k = 4.16$ in Equation 7.9b, for all porosities.

However, Macdonald et al. (1979) say that in Equation 7.9b, ε^3 should be replaced by $\varepsilon^{3.6}$, which is to say $k = 4.16/\varepsilon^{0.6}$. On the other hand, Meyer and Smith (1985) say that ε^3 in Equation 7.9b should be replaced by $\varepsilon^{4.1}$, which is to say, $k = 4.16/\varepsilon^{1.1}$. Indeed, Dullien (1979), reviewing the work of a dozen authors, suggests that the porosity function $\varepsilon^3/(1-\varepsilon)^2$ simply does not apply.

7.5 Other Aspects with Granular Media

Meyer and Smith (1985) conveniently provide data to consider. They sintered metal particles into disks using coarse particles to form some disks and fine particles to form others. With different forming pressures, they built 32 different disks with porosities ranging from 0.18 to 0.67 and examined them in three ways, by measuring

- Viscous permeability, B, m^2
- Porosity, ε
- The ratio of the area of pore walls to bulk volume, S, m^{-1}

They accomplished the third group of measurements by examining the thin disks under a microscope and measuring the perimeters of the pores. Considering that the disks have unit thickness, they arrived at S.

We now address a correlation between their values of B, ε, and S. From the above notations in Equation 7.2 the meaning of S is

$$\frac{1}{S} = \frac{V_o}{A_s} + \frac{V_s}{A_s} = \frac{V_o}{A_s} + \frac{V_o}{A_s}\frac{(1-\varepsilon)}{\varepsilon} \tag{7.13}$$

Since, in the text after Equation 7.3, V_o/A_s = the hydraulic diameter, d, we rewrite Equation 7.13 as Equation 7.14.

$$\frac{1}{S} = d + d\frac{(1-\varepsilon)}{\varepsilon} = d\left(1+\frac{1-\varepsilon}{\varepsilon}\right) \text{ or}$$

$$d = \frac{1}{S\left[1+\dfrac{1-\varepsilon}{\varepsilon}\right]} \tag{7.14}$$

From Equation 7.14, we deduce d from the values of S and ε provided by Meyer and Smith (1985). And we separately deduce d_F, the flow-average pore diameter, from Equation 7.8, using their values of B and ε. Then, on log/log paper, we plot d vs. d_F to see the correlation in Figure 7.2. Figure 7.2 shows that the ratio d/d_F is generally 0.30. Can we relate this ratio to the most probable pore-size distribution of Chapter 3? That is, can we relate it to the ratio of the number distribution to the fluid-flow distribution?

Consider the curves in Figure 7.3, which follow from Equation 3.3 where the scale factor, β equals 1.0. Curve A, a plot of Equation 7.15, shows the number distribution of pore diameters, X, in a layer of the medium. The most-popular diameter is $X = 1$ unit, the mean is $X = 2$.

$$f(X) = \frac{X}{\exp(X)} \tag{7.15}$$

Curve B, a plot of Equation 7.16, shows the distribution of fluid flow in that layer. The most popular pore diameter is $X = 4$ units, equal to the mean

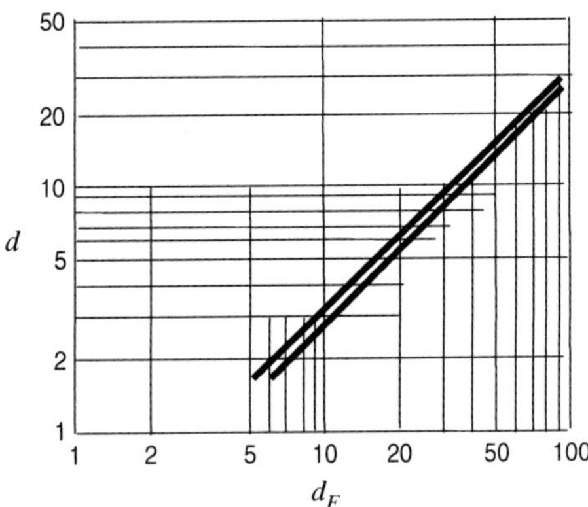

FIGURE 7.2
The correlation between d of Equation 7.14 and d_F of Equation 7.8 deduced from data of Meyer and Smith (1985) around sintered-particle disks. Between the two lines lie 32 points, evenly spread from one end to the other.

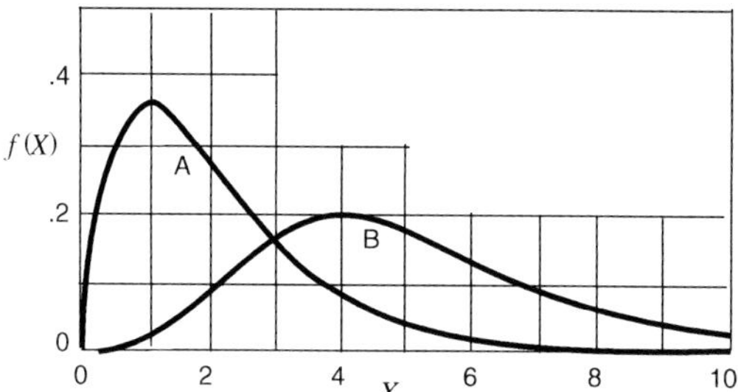

FIGURE 7.3
The most probable pore size distribution. Curve A, the number distribution of pore diameters, *X*, is a plot of Equation 7.15. Curve B, the viscous fluid flow distribution, is a plot of Equation 7.16.

when the fluid passes through many layers, recalling Figure 3.4. The mean flow pore diameter in a single layer is $X = 5$.

$$f(X) = \left[\frac{1}{24}\right]\frac{X^4}{\exp(X)} \tag{7.16}$$

Now consider the ratios of the most popular pore diameters in the two distributions: $1/4 = 0.25$. Then consider the ratios of the mean diameters: $2/5 = 0.40$. Does the above d/d_F ratio of 0.30 somehow correspond to the average of those ratios, $(0.25 + 0.40)/2 = 0.32$? Employing Math Model B of Chapter 3, instead of Model A, yields the same ratios. In any event, suppose we know *B* and ε and want to deduce S. After determining *dF* using Equation 7.8 and assuming the d/d_F ratio is 0.30, we can deduce *S* using

$$S = \frac{1}{0.30d_F\left[1 + \dfrac{1-\varepsilon}{\varepsilon}\right]} \tag{7.17}$$

8

Different Views of Filtration

8.1 Choosing Filter Media

Given a fluid, what filter medium should we use to use clarify it; to recover solids from it; or to sterilize it if it is otherwise particle free? Should we use a thick or thin filter medium? What flow-averaged pore diameter do we need? In classifying filter media as coarse, fine, in between, the arbitrary and often misleading micron rating has evolved. The micron rating, determined using a standardized filtration test, names the particle diameters stopped with great efficiency under the conditions of that test. As we saw in Chapter 6, however, there are many different ways of expressing filtration efficiency, and, of course, the rating changes when the tests conditions change.

The objective way to rate or classify a filter medium does not involve a filtration test; it involves the consideration of the following:

- Materials of construction
- Thickness
- Porosity, ratio of void volume to bulk volume
- Permeability, B in Chapter 1
- Porosity, whether one side is more porous than the other

Regarding the last point, usually the less porous side, the one with smaller pores, is faced downstream, in order to lengthen the life or increase the capacity of the medium. On the other hand, some media with very small pores in a thin layer on one side are designed to be used as a fine filter facing upstream, the other side being merely a coarser, thicker, and stronger support. But, in any case, when a manufacturer wants to sell his filter medium to a certain market, he must demonstrate the performance of his product by way of the specific standard filtration test for that market.

If an approved medium has passed a specific filtration test, another medium will pass the same test, provided it has the same five properties as the approved medium. Probably the most popular filtration test, and certainly one of the first with such detailed instructions, is the one specified by the National Fluid Power Association (NFPA) as the standard of that special field, ANSI/-NFPA T3.10.8.8 RI, now ISO Test 16889 (NFPA 1990). In the absence of other comparably detailed test procedures outside of that field, writers have used the language and views of the NFPA in addressing and defining the general field of liquid filtration. That is, many investigators have carried the thinking and the language of the NFPA procedure into areas where different thinking and different language are needed.

The American Society of Testing and Materials (ASTM) Committee F21, realizing that there can be no single standard filtration test for the great many different kinds of fluid streams, wrote three separate test procedures, one for a single pass at constant flow rate, Method F795, and one for a single pass at constant feed pressure, F796. And, since some members of the committee were familiar with the NFPA test, the committee wrote F797, a multipass test at constant flow-rate, in which, as in the NFPA procedure, the filtrate is returned to the feed tank where fresh test dust is constantly added.

But, these three ASTM procedures leave it to the investigator to choose the test liquid, the test particles, the velocity of fluid approaching the filter medium, and the temperature. Furthermore, the ASTM procedures leave it to the investigator to express filtration by either of the ways described in Chapter 6. The ASTM procedures, in essence, provide a checklist of what to look for in designing a filtration test. While the ASTM procedures are certainly not standard (since variations are considered), those procedures at least remind the investigator of how variations in conditions will change filtration efficiency, as well as the different meanings of filtration efficiency. A review of the different fields of filtration follows in the next section.

8.2   Views of the NFPA and the SAE

A manufacturer of hydraulic power equipment or of gasoline or diesel engines approaches a producer of filter cartridges (also called elements) with requirements for filtering hydraulic fluid, lubrication oil, or fuel oil. The cartridge must handle a certain constant volumetric flow rate and fit into certain housing. To test the cartridge, place it in a test stand. Using a positive-displacement pump, feed a specific oil stream, containing test dust, at a constant flow rate. The driving pressure rises with time. Periodically take samples of the feed and filtrate streams for analysis. Stop the test when the driving pressure reaches some upper limit.

The cartridge manufacturer, after designing and testing the cartridge according to specific NFPA or Society of Automotive Engineers (SAE) procedures, reports that it can supply a cartridge that demonstrates certain Beta ratios (Section 6.3) at separating test dust from the oil and that a certain mass of test dust can be fed to the cartridge before the driving pressure reaches an upper limit.

The manufacturer must design a cartridge that is both efficient and long lived, not to mention inexpensive and rugged. The manufacturer must provide the results of a multipass filtration test where the filtrate is returned to the feed tank and fresh test dust is continuously added to the feed tank to maintain a constant concentration of test particles in the feed stream. But constant concentration refers to the mass concentration of test dust. Over time, the feed stream becomes richer in the number of small particles, which are not separated with the efficiency of large particles and have relatively little mass. Thus, the composition of the feed stream is not really constant.

While NFPA and SAE test procedures specify the temperature, viscosity, and electrical properties of the oil, the filter manufacturer knows that the lower the approach velocity of the oil through the filter medium, the greater the filtration efficiency. Thus, in his cartridge, he crowds in as much filter surface area as he can, in the form of a pleated paper filter medium.

8.3   Views in the Chemical Process Industry

In that wide arena called the chemical process industry, the filter manufacturer is not so restricted in providing the best surface area of the filter medium. That is, for a given sized stream to be filtered with a content of specific solids, the filter manufacture will recommend either the best number of cartridges or bags or the best area of a filter cloth to be used in a plate-and-frame filter or in a continuous-belt filter. If the solids are the material to be recovered, the filter cloth must release those solids easily. In conducting a filtration test, the filter manufacturer or the user will employ actual samples of the process stream. The tests can be quite simple — a single pass, constant pressure or vacuum test on a lab bench — or elaborate — with pumps and other equipment. The characteristics to look for are:

- Filtration efficiency as a function of fluid velocity at a specific temperature or perhaps at different temperatures to address summer versus winter conditions
- Capacity of the medium as to how soon it plugs with accumulated solids or forms a certain depth of filter cake
- Ease of backwashing and reusing the medium

The filter manufacturer may have to recommend a two-stage process: one filter medium and then another. Or perhaps, when recovering solids is not the aim, the first stage may involve the use of a filter aid, while the second stage may involve mere polishing of the liquid. Indeed, the second stage may require a medium that stops test microbes, a matter we address later. Alternatively, the polishing filter medium, such as used in the electronics industry, may be required to stop very fine mineral particles, while at the same time not adding soluble material to the filtrate. And the medium must be resistant to the harsh fluids involved.

The filter medium may be required to clarify a gas stream by separating very small particles, including microbes. The filter medium may be a bed of sand. The filter medium may have to be heat resistant, as are metal fibers used to withstand molten polymers or a heat resistant cloth used to clarify stack gases.

8.4   Views in Cross-Flow Filtration

So far, we have discussed dead end filtration. In many liquid filtration problems it is advantageous to employ cross-flow filtration (Chapter 12). Here the feed stream runs over the face of the filter medium at high velocities as one portion of the stream passes through the medium while the other portion sweeps away solids that would otherwise collect on and plug the medium.

But even here the medium has a finite life, although sometimes it can be backwashed and used again for a limited number of cycles. This scheme requires balancing the portion of the feed stream that passes through the medium against the portion that does not. That which does not pass through is recirculated back to the source of the feed stream or treated in another fashion. When the filter medium is a very fine membrane or a bundle of microporous tubes (hollow fibers), even soluble materials are separated from the liquid, such as high molecular weight compounds.

8.5   Separating Immiscible Fluids

In some situations, a liquid to be filtered contains droplets of another, immiscible liquid — for example, water in oil or vice versa. In other situations, a gas to be filtered contains droplets of a liquid. Further, in all these cases, solid particles are also suspended in the fluid to be filtered, making the separation more difficult.

8.6 Filtration Testing Guidelines

Keep the following points in mind when designing or performing a filtration test:

- While the use of given test particles and a given test fluid at a given velocity, often viewed as the given driving pressure, will give the investigator data to rate a filter medium, the use of the real fluid, with its real particles, will yield different test results.

- When sorting out filter media to test, consider the properties mentioned in Section 8.1, and the rules of thumb discussed in the last portion of Section 6.3.

9

Filtering Liquids

9.1 General Principles

If a liquid contains no droplets of an immiscible liquid but only suspended particles and if we have no need to recover the particles to be separated, the following generalizations apply. As particles approach the face of a filter medium, those particles larger than the pores do not enter. Those that do enter the few large pores do not get very far. Recall the probability curves in Figure 3.4. As medium-sized particles enter the face of the filter medium, some may go deep into it, and some may even pass through. Some that do not pass through pull away from the laminar flow stream as the stream turns a corner so that inertia carries them to a pore wall. Once on the wall they stick, by van der Waals forces, unless knocked off by sudden surges in fluid flow or vibration. In laminar flow the velocity of the liquid on the pore wall is nil, so the particles are not easily washed away.

On the other hand, small particles tend to stay in the laminar stream. In laminar pipe flow, particles concentrate in the center of the pipe. But small particles exhibit more Brownian motion than large particles. Thus there is a statistical chance that some small particles, in their random movements, will find themselves up against a pore wall. The hotter the temperature, the less viscous the carrier fluid; and the smaller the particles, the more Brownian movement. Furthermore, small particles may be attracted to the pore walls by differences in the zeta potential of the particle and the wall (Section 1.10 and Section 9.2). And the lower the velocity of the carrier fluid or the thicker the filter medium, the more time particles have to randomly break out of the laminar stream and hit a pore wall. Thus, given a certain filter medium, we can more efficiently clarify a mobile liquid than a viscous one. And we can more easily clarify a gas than a liquid because of the low viscosity of gasses.

9.2   Zeta Potential

We continue the discussion of zeta potential that began in Section 1.10. At a solid-liquid or liquid-liquid interface, a collection of positive and negative charges form on the surface of the solid or on suspended liquid droplets. This double layer is made up of ions in aqueous solution that are held firmly to the surface and float in a more diffuse, mobile layer extending into the solution.

The resulting net charge of the diffuse layer is equal in magnitude but opposite in sign to that of the firmly held or fixed layer. Because of these electrical charges, there exists a difference in potential between the fixed layers and the bulk of the solution. This is called the electrokinetic potential or the zeta potential. If the zeta potential of a particle in suspension is opposite in sign to the zeta potential of the pore walls in a filter medium, the particles will be attracted to the wall. Recall Cohn's Law relating zeta potentials to dielectric constants. For example, water has a dielectric constant of 70, greater than cellulose fibers, 5. Hence, by Cohn's Law, cellulose fibers, in water, have a negative zeta potential. Quartz (silica) has a dielectric constant of 4, also less than water, and hence also has a negative zeta potential in water. Titanate fibers have a dielectric constant of about 14,000 and thus a positive zeta potential in water. That is why those fibers are mixed with cellulose fibers in forming a filter medium. Jaisinghani and Verdegan (1982) describe how to measure the zeta potential of a filter medium.

9.2.1   Examples of Zeta Potential

From Cohn's Law we know that when we filter silica test dust from water by means of a bed of cellulose fibers, silica particles are not attracted to the fibers. But when we coat the fibers with, for example, a polyamine, we change the sign of the zeta potential. The results of a filter medium so treated show a dramatic increase in the efficiency with which it captures silica particles (e.g., Cuno's Zeta Plus™ filter media).

A coarse medium with a polyamine coating can filter as a fine medium. The coating does not change the permeability of the medium. For a given flow of water through the medium, the addition of the coating does not mean we must apply a greater driving pressure to obtain the same flow without the coating. But we must be aware of the following:

- When we use a fine grade medium without a polyamine coating in an extended filtration run, we notice that filtration efficiency usually increases as the pores become clogged with the captured particles. We stop the run when the resistance increases to an unacceptable level.

- When we use a coarse medium with a polyamine coating that enables the medium to filter as efficiently as the fine medium, we notice that before we see a rise in resistance, filtration efficiency drops. Particles attracted to the pore walls neutralize the zeta potential of the walls and capture efficiency drops as other particles come along.

This is not to say we should avoid the advantage of coated fibers. Where we would need a given driving pressure to get a certain flow rate with an uncoated fine medium, switching to a coated coarse medium enables us to enjoy the same filtration efficiency but with as little as $1/_{10}$ the driving pressure. This advantage is useful when the liquid is very viscous. But we must know when to stop the run. We must know from tests beforehand the electrical capacity of the medium, or we must monitor the filtrate.

9.3 Sieving Filtration.

Apart from the impact of zeta potentials on filtration efficiency or the chance that a particle smaller than a pore may find a pore wall, one goal in filtration is simply to use a filter medium with pores small enough to stop particle sizes of interest. Whether the length of the average pore is a hundred or a thousand times the average particle diameter; we just want our filter medium to have a small flow-averaged pore diameter. We want a filter medium in which the largest pores are small enough. That way we will stop particle sizes of interest, regardless of the viscosity or velocity of the liquid.

A sieve is a thin material with straight-through pores that are all the same size. A sieve stops all particles larger than its openings and, in the absence of any zeta-potential actions, passes all particles smaller than its openings. But writers speak of sieving filtration with microporous membranes without meaning the track-etched type.

We begin by recalling the most probable pore-size distribution, Math Model A, in Chapter 3. Equation 9.1 describes laminar-flow pore distribution in a thin layer of a filter medium where pore diameters, X units, are larger than, or certainly not smaller than, the thickness.

$$f(X) = \frac{1}{24} \frac{X^4}{\exp(X)} \tag{9.1}$$

Figure 9.1 shows two plots of this equation. The notation $F(X)$ means cumulative volume of fluid flow liquid, in contrast to $f(X)$, the volumetric flow through different sized pores. When particles of diameter 2 units approach the medium, most of them will pass through the larger pores; only

10% will approach pores that size or smaller. Thus 2-diameter particles will be stopped with an efficiency of 0.10. Continuing with that logic, the $F(X)$ curve in Figure 9.1 shows the efficiency with which particles of different sizes are stopped. Now recall the kind of graph paper used in Figure 6.2. Onto that graph paper are drawn the cumulative, $F(X)$ curve of Figure 9.1 to yield Figure 9.2. Notice the slope, measured using the ratio of the right vertical scale to the horizontal scale. It is somewhat greater than 2.0.

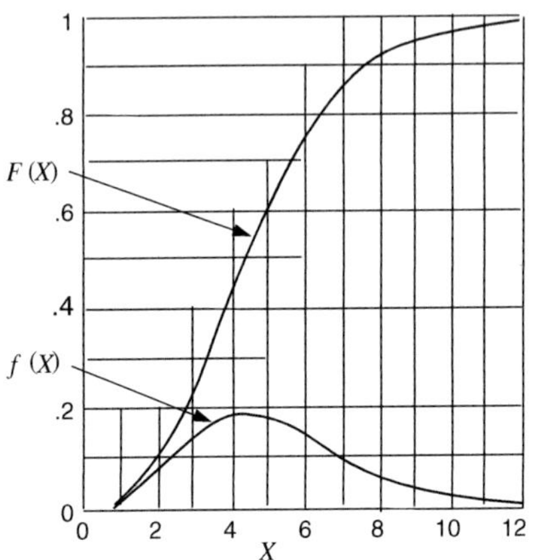

FIGURE 9.1
Plots of Equation 9.1.

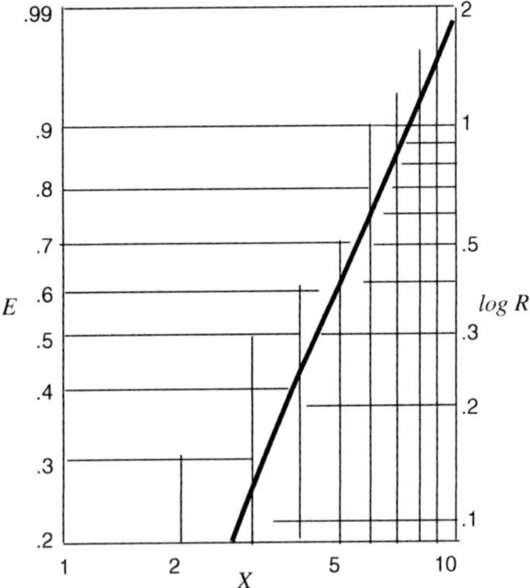

FIGURE 9.2
Employing the $F(X)$ curve in Figure 9.1 to predict the filtration efficiencies, E, of X-diameter particles.

As illustrated in Figure 3.4, when a fluid passes through 10 such layers, the flow-pore distribution becomes narrow. In that case, a plot like Figure 9.2 would show a curve with a slope much greater than 2.0 Now recall the experimental filtration results in Figure 6.4. Even the steepest curve, C, with a slope of 1.6, is far from showing sieving filtration. Some small particles passing through large pores do indeed find a pore wall and stick.

9.4 Another View of Sieving Filtration

Grant and Zahka (1990) provide data on sieving filtration. Over the course of many experiments, Grant (1988) fed distilled water suspensions of twelve different sized spheres, diameters from 0.12 to 0.55 μm, to three different membranes rated at 0.1, 0.2, and 0.45 μm. He determined the log reduction values, R, of different sized spheres for each of the three different membranes. His results, plotted in Figure 9.3 are straight lines with slopes of 1.48. However, Grant's meaning of sieving differs from the meaning in Section 9.3. To Grant, sieving means normal filtration. He takes into account all the variables associated with such a separation, which he calls particle removal mechanisms. Grant offers a mathematical model of R values expected considering many variables. This writer makes no attempt to explain that model;

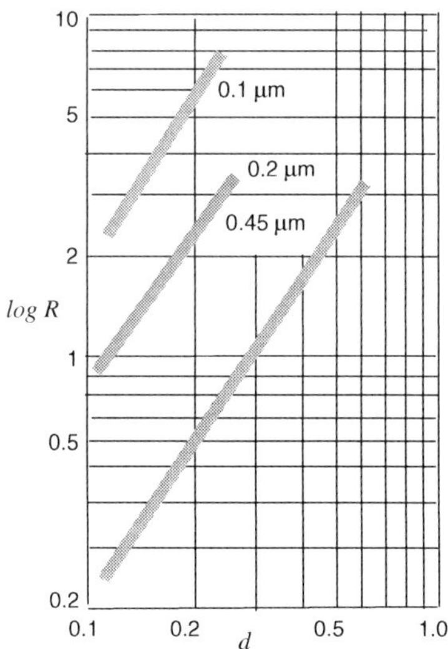

FIGURE 9.3
Filtration efficiencies expressed as *log R* values of *d*-diameter, μm, particles by three differently rated microporous membranes. (From Grant and Zahka 1990).

however, some idea of the model is obtained through the following excerpt of Grants' writings.

> The model predicts the [filtration ratio of given-sized particles] from the initial reduced dimensionless filter coefficient, the flow redistribution parameter, [and] the number of pore volumes of fluid passed through the filter media…. The flow rate through each pore is proportional to the volume of the pores…. [The flow redistribution parameter] characterizes the way in which the flow paths through the media are redistributed as pores within the media become clogged with particles.

Grant's model predicts that with continued filtration and the feeding of more particles, the filtration ratio falls as particles break through. For example, an initial log R value drops from 6 to 3 after 0.005 pore volumes of particles have been removed, after which the log R values level off. The phrase in quotes apparently refers to the fact that after the membrane has been fed a certain volume of particles — a volume corresponding to 0.005 of the volume of pores — filtration reaches a more or less steady state condition within the time studied as reflected in Figure 9.2. Grant implies that, during this time, the very small pores become clogged with collected particles, after which the flow stream is directed to larger pores, which allow particles through that would have been otherwise stopped by the small pores. That is, no neutralizing of zeta potentials occurs, as discussed in Section 9.2.1.

In another example, Sueoka and Malchesky (1983) used ultrafilter membranes to stop Angstrom-sized molecules of dextran and blood components. They plotted filtration efficiency (rejection) on a probability scale vs. molecular size on a log scale. That is, they used the same chart paper as in Figure 3.1. They obtained straight lines, implying log-normal distributions of flow-pore diameters with geometric standard deviations ranging from 1.51 to 2.13.

9.5 Absolute Filtration

An implied definition of absolute filtration is provided by ASTM D3862 and ASTM D3863. These test procedures use a 47-mm-diameter disk of a microporous membrane with a surface area of 10 cm². A 100-ml broth containing 10^8 freshly grown test microbes is placed on top of the membrane and then sucked through into a flask below (vacuum level not specified), after which live microbes in the filtrate are counted. When this filtrate is found to be sterile, the membrane is considered absolute at stopping microbes of that size. That is, if the microbe is *Serratia marcescens*, the membrane is rated as 0.45 µm. Of course, absolute means a log-reduction value of greater than 8. When a single microbe is found in the filtrate, the log reduction value is indeed 8. The filtration efficiency is 0.999 999 99. Remember, the definition of heat sterilization is a log-reduction value of 6: a kill efficiency of 0.999 999.

Some investigators, attempting to demonstrate that a membrane is indeed absolute at stopping microbes of a certain size, challenge a cartridge containing 4500 cm^2 of membrane surface with a broth containing 10^{12} microbes ($2.2 \cdot 10^8$ microbes per cm^2). When they find one telltale microbe in the filtrate, they proclaim that the cartridge failed the challenge test. Yet, even if they had found 200 microbes in the filtrate, they would still have demonstrated a log reduction value greater than 7 per cm^2, the original premise for absolute filtration. As a practical matter, membranes used in the pharmaceutical industry are never challenged with such enormous numbers of microbes. Indeed, Vavorsky (2003) explains that before the final sterile filtration step, a liquid is prefiltered and, before that, clarified in other separation steps.

9.6 Inferring Pore Sizes from Filtration Tests

Do not attempt to infer pore sizes from filtration tests. Consider two filter media, each composed of the same material(s), each with the same porosity and permeability and, thus, the same pore-size distribution. But one is thicker than the other. The thicker material will be the more efficient filter, in which case some investigators will conclude that the thick medium has smaller pores. Recall Grant's data in Figure 9.3. A membrane rated as 0.45 μm stopped 0.45-μm-diameter latex spheres with a log R value of only 2. Johnston (1975) found that the same size particles of black iron oxide were also stopped with a log R value near 2.

9.7 Reaching a Standard by Which to Rate Media

We hope the reader understands by now that there is no such thing as a universal standard liquid-filtration test. To be sure, many different so-called standard tests exist, each one intended to rate media for a specific application. Indeed, many filtration tests apply a pore-size rating, which, in the light of Section 9.6, is meaningless. Nonetheless, since many users of filter media have grown accustomed to such pore-size ratings, the filter manufacturer is forced to tack this meaningless label onto his product.

For example, Alderete (1991), showing the results of filtration tests under specific conditions (Arizona road dust in water at a specific temperature and flow rate) of different cartridges, explains nominal, absolute, and Beta ratings. But he also points out that under different conditions these tests would yield different results. Many filter users, however, without the time to consider the many ramifications of filtration, only want to hear the rating. But at least the producers of membranes, who have been forced to rate their products by pore size, provide more information about their products than do producers of other filter media. Membrane producers provide useful information, reporting:

- Material(s) of construction
- Thickness
- Porosity
- Data on fluid flow-rate vs. pressure drop
- Whether the material is homogeneous or has one side denser than the other

Because a rating, based on a single standard filtration test, is specious, the truly informative investigator addresses all five of these issues when describing and evaluating a filter medium. This author recalls a meeting where the speaker, describing a resin-impregnated filter paper, reported such information as basis weight and caliper but when asked about porosity essentially answered, "What has that got to do with anything?"

Of course, if we knew the density of the fibers with their resin coating we could infer porosity from the basis weight (mass per area) and the caliper (thickness). Or in the case of a non-woven cloth like polyester, we could also infer porosity from basis weight and caliber, knowing the density of polyester. Manufacturers of filter paper and nonwoven cloths will do filtration customers a favor if they report porosity straight away, along with thickness and permeability (Chapter 1 and Chapter 2). Some writers and speakers confuse porosity with pore size. Chapter 11 says more about the ratings of microporous meant for sterilization filtration.

9.8   Filter Media Composed of Nanofibers

Suthar and Chase (2002) describe the results of liquid filtration tests on media composed of plastic fibers with diameters in the nanometer range. They performed filtration tests on media built of ordinary-diameter fibers (175 μm), then tested media with added fibers of diameters less than 1 μm. As expected, they found the latter combination to be more efficient at stopping masses of TiO_2 particles. While the authors report such data as permeability, the relative masses of nanofibers to ordinary ones, and assert that all media were of equal thickness, they do not report the porosities of the media.

If we knew the porosities we could infer the flow-averaged pore diameter using Equation 1.7 and then relate that to filtration efficiency. Using Equation

7.14, we could estimate the internal surface area, provided, of course, that the liquid permeability measurements were in the laminar-flow range.

Gas flow measurements of permeability cannot be used in such calculation because gas flows around nanofibers are diluted with Knudsen flow.

While Suthar and Chase do indeed report the masses of the different-sized fibers, it would have been helpful if they had also estimated the relative surface area of the different fibers. After all, filtration efficiency is a function of both pore size and internal surface area as well as zeta potentials and residence times.

Tepper et al. (2002) employed nanofibers of alumina into (on top of?) media of cellulose and glass. Such mixtures stopped viruses. Furthermore, the permeabilities of their mixtures were 10 times those of microporous membranes designed to do the job. They suggest that alumina nanofibers could replace asbestos nanofibers now banned in pharmaceutical filtrations.

10

Filtering Gasses

10.1 Gas Filtration and Liquid Filtration Compared

Gas filtration differs from liquid filtration in three respects:

1. In gas filtration, particle diameters in the range of 0.1 to 0.5 µm are separated with the least efficiency; that is, both larger and smaller particles are stopped with greater efficiency. Apparently no one has seen or predicted this in liquid filtration. Indeed, particle-sensing instruments for examining liquids are not available for detecting particle diameters smaller than about 0.5 µm.

2. A mathematical model of gas filtration successfully predicts the efficiency with which a single fiber collects particles, in viscous flow, without Knudsen flow (Liu and Rubow 1986). This model considers the three mechanisms of particle capture: direct interception, inertia, and Brownian diffusion. It includes the diameter of the fiber, the diameters of the particles, and the velocity of the gas. Yet a velocity that is too low or too high negatively affects particle capture (Jaroszczyk and Wake 1991).

3. It follows, then, that the overall efficiency with which a fibrous bed collects particles becomes a function of the number of fibers in the bed, or, more specifically, the total area of the fiber surfaces encountered by a unit volume of the gas.

Recall Equation 7.11 and Equation 7.12, relating permeability to fiber diameter and porosity. From those expressions we can deduce the internal surface area of the bed. And, for a granular medium, recall Equation 7.14 and Equation 7.17, which also relate the internal area to permeability and porosity.

The only pore model for filtration efficiency that can be applied in gas filtration is the one that describes a particular medium: the track-etched membrane with equal-diameter straight-through tunnels. The performance of the other types of membranes, produced by the solvent-cast method, fit the fiber surface area model (Liu and Rubow 1986).

Thus with these gas-filtration models at hand, we may deduce the best filter medium for a given gas stream. Not so in liquid filtration, where we must make test runs to select the best medium.

However, gas filtration is similar to liquid filtration in at least three ways:

1. The filtration model can include electrical aspects (Trottier and Brown 1990). We may electronically enhance a gas filter by including a resin with the fibers (Davies 1973). The resin, a nonconductor, readily acquires a static charge to capture particles (akin, in liquid filtration, to altering the zeta potential). Or, we can pass the gas-feed stream though a screen electrode just before the filter medium, while on the downstream side of the medium hold another electrode in place. A high voltage applied across the electrodes greatly enhances the filtration efficiency (VanOsdell and Donovan 1986).

2. A gas filter medium has a finite capacity, called effectiveness — the mass of particles collected per unit face area before a significant drop in permeability (not to be confused with the other code word, arrestance, referring to filtration efficiency). Yet often, as in a bag-house, designed to clarify various exhaust gases, the medium, the bags, can be shaken free of particles or back-blasted, and used again for many numbers of cycles.

3. Writers express filtration efficiency in the two different ways of Figure 6.2 and also as total mass efficiency or cumulative mass efficiency with decreasing particle diameters.

10.2 Test Methods in Gas Filtration

A test stand for gas filtration — usually air filtration — is more complicated than a test stand for liquid filtration. The air must be kept at a constant temperature and humidity; it must approach the filter medium evenly, at a specific velocity; and the test particles must be suspended in the air stream as homogeneously as possible. The test stand gets more complicated when we consider what test particles to use, how to generate them, how to suspend them in the air stream, how to count them, and how to compare the particle-size distribution in the feed stream to that in the filtrate.

Often we do not look at the particle-size distribution, we simply consider the total mass of particles in the two streams. For example, a known mass of fine grade Arizona road dust is fed to the medium; then the medium is weighed to find the increase in mass. Here we learn what fraction of the mass of the feed stream dust has been arrested by the filter. Jaroszczyk (1987a) describes a device for feeding test dust.

Alternatively, the dust is premixed with carbon black and lint, and during the run, samples of both feed and filtrate streams are passed through an analytical filter to compare the degrees of staining.

Powdered alumina, with a mass-median particle diameter of 5.2 μm, has been used as test particles.

Dyes such as methylene blue, with a mass-median diameter of 0.5 μm, and uranin, with a mass-median diameter of 0.2 μm, have been used as test aerosols. Samples of the air streams are passed through an analytical filter, which is then examined for the degree of coloring.

Low-vapor-pressure oils have been converted into aerosols. Pierce et al. measured the efficiency up to 0.99999 with which a medium stops individual droplets of diameters ranging from 0.07 to 0.3 μm. They examined air streams with a condensation nucleus counter.

Latex spheres, freed from aqueous suspension and dispersed in air by means of a special device, have been used as test aerosols. An optical particle counter examines the air streams (ASTM F1215).

Particles of NaCl have been used in diameters ranging from 0.001 to 1.0 μm. The sizes are measured with a differential mobility particle sizer. In this case the air streams are examined with a laser diode detector or a flame ionization detector (Simpson and Iverson 1989). Of course, the size of the test particles to use depends on the size of the particles one wants to demonstrate that the filter will arrest.

More details on the kinds of test procedures just discussed are provided in *STP 975* (ASTM 1986). See also Jaroszczyk and Ptak (1985); Jaroszczyk (1987a, 1987b); Edward Johnson et al. (1990); Brian Johnson et al. (1990); and Remiarz et al.

A special kind of air filter called a vent filter is used in the pharmaceutical industry. It is a pleated membrane cartridge placed over a tank. A vent filter allows air in or out of the tank as it is filled with liquid or drained but prevents the passage of microbes. The membrane, which has a pretested bubble point high enough to stop microbes, is made of a hydrophobic material and kept hot with a steam jacket to prevent condensation of water vapor within the pores. Another kind of air filter used in the pharmaceutical industry is a glass fiber mat designed to filter air fed to fermenters. It is pretested with an aerosol of corn oil (Meltzer 1987). Dickenson (1992) provides many illustrations of gas filtration media and systems.

10.3 Filter Media with Nanofibers

Graham et al. (2002) describe a medium composed of nanodiameter plastic fibers deposited on the face of an ordinary mat of plastic fibers. Addition of the nanofibers increased gas filtration efficiency without a drop in permeability.

Furthermore, the medium could be reused after cyclic air pulse jet back cleaning.

Nanofibers are more efficient than larger fibers in collecting particles because air does not flow around nanofibers in laminar flow. That is, in laminar flow the velocity of a liquid over the very surface is nil. But when fiber diameters are smaller than the mean free path of gas molecules, a finite velocity of gas directly flows across the surfaces of the nanofibers, thereby more efficiently carrying particles to those surfaces, where they stick. The authors show a picture of NaCl particles stuck like Christmas tree ornaments on nanofibers.

11

The Rating of a Membrane Filter Medium

11.1 Revisiting Elford (1933)

Presented with the filtration results in Figure 6.4, of how a single filter paper performs under different conditions, how then do we come up with a performance rating? Obviously we cannot, since performance depends on the conditions of filtration. The only objective way to rate the filter paper is to address five properties (previously mentioned in Chapter 8):

- Material(s) of construction
- Porosity
- Permeability
- Thickness
- Whether one face is more porous than the other

The same is true of microporous membranes, Producers of microporous membranes, in essence, address these five points more than producers of paper or other nonwoven fibrous media. Yet users of membrane filters and governmenfal agencies want assurances that, in spite of variations in filtration conditions, a certain size microbe will indeed be stopped with great efficiency. This demand leads to the simple reasoning: build the membrane with pores smaller than the size of the microbes of interest. Then, these questions arise: What filtration efficiency is high enough? and What size microbes are of interest?

To address these questions, consider the experimental results reported by Elford (1933), depicted in Figure 11.1 (a tracing of Elford's Figure 7). Elford shows, in four separate filtration tests, the increasing efficiencies with which membranes with decreasing pore diameters stop *B. prodigiosus*, now known as *Serratia marcescens*. That is, with a pore diameter of 1.5 μm, the filtrate was sterile only if less than 10^4 microbes were fed to the membrane, which was a small-diameter disk. Yet with a pore diameter of 0.9 μm, 10^8 microbes were stopped. Putting aside for the moment the question of what Elford

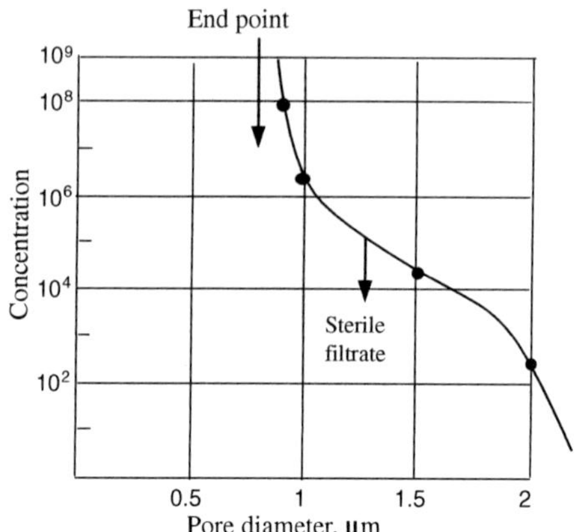

FIGURE 11.1

A tracing of Elford's 1933 Figure 7, illustrating the decreasing pore diameter in microporous membranes to provide a sterile filtrate from broths of a test microbe with increasing concentration. Apparently concentration refers to the numbers of microbes fed per unit surface area of the membranes. Elford refers to the critical small diameter as the end point. The test microbe is *B. prodigiosus*. Elford, in reporting pore diameters, refers to a previous paper for the method of measurement. The present writer, not having seen that paper, but assuming that pore diameter correspond to the reciprocal of the bubble point, makes the plot in Figure 11.2.

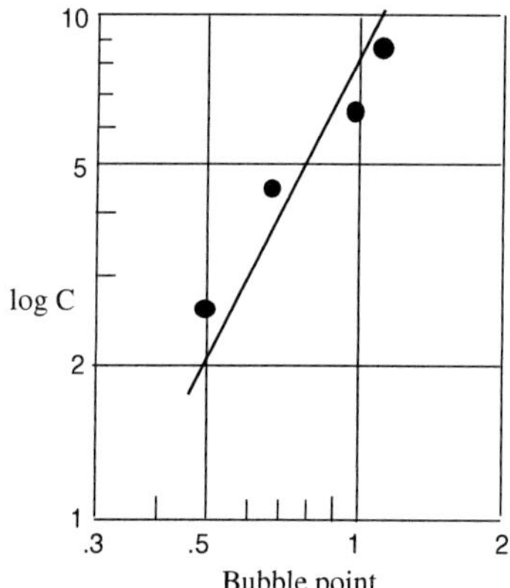

FIGURE 11.2

An alternative plot on log/log paper of data in Figure 11.1. Here bubble point is the simple reciprocal of pore diameter (Figure 4.1), in arbitrary units. "C" is Elford's concentration treated as the filtration ratio R (Section 6.3).

meant by pore diameter, which Elford addressed in a previous paper not seen by the present writer, the subject to focus on in Figure 11.1 is Elford's concept of the end point. It refers to the pore diameter small enough to stop all such test microbes. We now replot Elford's data on log/log paper. Since we know that the bubble point corresponds to the reciprocal of the pore diameter (Section 4.1), we plot, in Figure 11.2, the log of Elford's C (on a log scale) vs. bubble point. The four points describe a straight line with a slope of 2.0.

Johnston and Meltzer (1979), showing such a plot, also plotted the results of Reti (1977), showing log R (Section 6.3) vs. bubble point, and of Pall and Kirnbauer (1978), to also see lines with slopes of 2.0. And, when they plotted the many results of Leahy and Sullivan (1978), on the same graph paper, the slope was also 2.0. Moreover, Reti's (1977) results, employing two different fluid-driving pressures, also showed the same slopes. Yet with one pressure 10 times that of the other (meaning fluid-residence times $^1/_{10}$ the other) log R values of the shorter residence times were about 0.7 those of the longer residence times. Which is to say, the clear end point of which Elford speaks does not exist. We must come to grips with a filtration efficiency, expressed as log R, that is "Enough, already!"

Once having addressed that question, investigators have rated a membrane by the diameter of the test microbe stopped with that great efficiency. Which is to say, given a certain thickness of a membrane and a certain fluid-driving pressure, we employ a membrane with high enough bubble points to stop 10^7 microbes presented to each square centimeter of the membrane.

11.2 Test Microbes Used

Listed in Table 11.1 are the different test microbes used to arrive at ratings. Elford (1933) reports that 0.5–1.0 μm is the diameter of *B. prodigiosus* (*Serratia marcescens*). Modern photographs show the rod shape. It then seemed to have followed that a membrane to stop that microbe with high efficiency is rated as 0.45 μm pore size. Such membranes were then used as sterilizing filters. Then investigators found other microbes in filtrates. Those microbes were cultured as *Pseudomonas diminuta* (now called *Brevundimonas diminuta*). It followed that a membrane to stop those microbes must have a smaller rating, hence the rating of 0.20 μm (or 0.22 μm).

However, the diameters of these smaller microbes are not half those of the previous microbes. Leahy and Sullivan (1978) show photographs of the rod-shaped *P. diminuta* (copied by Meltzer 1987). The diameter is 0.49 μm and the length is 1.3 μm. Where does the 0.20 (or 0.22) rating come from? Perhaps these separate microbes have different surface charges, akin to or the same as zeta potentials. Which is to say, for a given membrane material one microbe is captured more efficiently than the other. Indeed, Trotter at al. (2002) report that different membrane materials show different efficiencies of capturing a given microbe.

TABLE 11.1

Test Microbes Used to Rate Membranes

Membrane Rating, μm	Test Microbe
0.65–0.8	Saccharomyces cereviseae
0.45	Serratia marcescens
0.30	Pseudomonas aeriginosa
0.22	Pseudomonas diminuta
0.10	Acholeplasma species

Source: From Bower (1986).

11.3 Filtration Efficiency Required of Test Microbes

Meltzer (1987) reports that membrane manufacturers, meeting under the aegis of the Health Manufacturing Association, defined a sterilizing membrane as a membrane that would stop 10^7 *P. diminuta* for each square centimeter of area under a fluid-driving pressure of 30 psi (2 bars). But how much of the membrane surface will be covered by those microbes? To answer that, consider that a square centimeter consists of 10^8 μm². A single *P. diminuta* casts a shadow of $0.49 \times 1.2 = 0.59$ μm², so that 10^7 of them will cast a shadow of 0.59×10^7 μm². Thus, $0.59 \cdot 10^7 / 10^8 = 0.059$ of the membrane surface will be covered, if no microbes are on top of one another.

Writers who say that these numbers of microbes will be sufficient to find the oversize pores as if the membrane were a thin sieve have not thought it through. To do what they want requires at least 1.7×10^8 *P. diminuta* per square centimeter. Or if only the surface pores, which constitute about 0.75 of the surface area, are to be covered, then 1.3×10^8 microbes approach the job. However, the microbes will fall on random spots. That is, from the Poisson distribution (the discrete form of the continuous gamma distribution, Johnston 1999b), with the mean at 1.0 microbe per unit area, we expect that 36% of the unit areas will remain empty, another 36% will hold a single microbe, as the remaining areas will hold two or more microbes. Although this line of inquiry may be tedious, we must consider another tedious question. If 10^8 test microbes are fed to 10 cm² of membrane surface, and one microbe appears in the filtrate, does the membrane pass the test? Yes, because less than one microbe passed 1 cm² fed 10^7 microbes.

Now consider a question posed by Wallhäusser (1979). First, we describe what he did. To each of four different 0.20-μm-rated filter cartridges from four different manufacturers he fed 21 liters of a stream containing 10^9 *P. diminuta* per liter. He sampled 1-liter portions of the filtrates to find from 1 to 100 microbes per liter. He then asked the question: Were these cartridges, each with 4500 cm² of membrane surface, effective in sterilizing those streams?

Johnston and Meltzer (1979) answered that question by pointing out that the results did indeed meet the test of stopping at least 10^7 microbes per square centimeter of membrane surface. Moreover, no one cartridge was any more efficient in stopping microbes than the others.

Yet membranes of different materials but of equal ratings perform differently. Trotter et al. (2002) demonstrated the rule of thumb (Section 6.3) saying that by increasing the thickness of a filter medium by a factor of two, log R values increase by the same factor. They employed two 0.45-μm-rated membranes in series and stopped *B. diminuta* with the same efficiency as a single 0.20-μm-rated membrane. They tested membranes of four different materials and overwhelmed the membranes with microbes. To what look like 3.9-cm² disks they fed a 300-mL broth of *B. diminuta*, containing a count of 10^7 per mL. That is, they fed 10^9 microbes to each square centimeter. They then fed that filtrate to a second 0.45-μm-rated membrane. And they employed two different driving pressures, 5 and 30 psi.

They saw no different results between the two driving pressures. But, the log R values after the first filters varied from 2.0 to 8.3 and from the second filters varied from 0.85 to 3.35, for total log R values ranging from 2.85 to 9.5. In descending order of performance (highest log R values first) the materials were polyamide, poly(ether sulfone), cellulose acetate, and poly(vinylidene diflouride). We would expect membranes of different materials to perform differently. Yet we do not know how they were rated, which raises the question: Did all membranes of equal ratings but of different materials have equal flow-averaged pore diameters and thicknesses? If so, then we fall back on the question of performance: If, by definition, a 0.20-μm-rated membrane must stop *B. diminuta* with great efficiency, then the flow-averaged pore diameter must be adjusted for the material of the membrane. That is, the flow-averaged pore diameter of the poly(vinylidene diflouride) membrane must be less than that of the polyamide membrane.

Trotter et al. (2002) mention a recommendation of the Federal Drug Administration (FDA) implying that when viscous fluids are involved, two such membranes should be used, with the extra surface area, to better absorb the bio-burden. Of course, the total pressure drop of a clean fluid across two 0.45-μm-rated membranes is about the same as across a single 0.20-μm-rated membrane. However, Yavorsky (2002) suggests separating the bio-burden with less expensive depth filter media, before the final membrane filter.

11.4 Properties of Membranes vs. Ratings

With this is mind, consider data reported by an early provider of membranes. The Millipore Corporation, in their Catalogue MC/1, 1971, lists the properties of their membrane filters vs. ratings. That is, they report air and water flow rates vs. driving pressure vs. ratings (partly addressed in Figure 2.3). They also

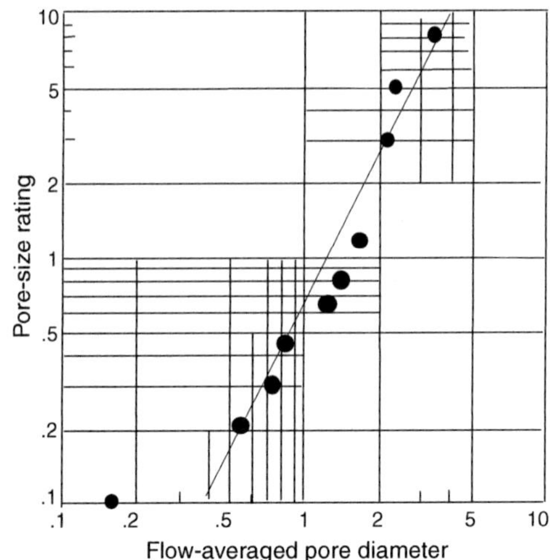

FIGURE 11.3
Plot of data deduced from properties of cellulose-ester membrane as reported by the producer, the Millipore Corporation. Units of measure expressed in micrometers. The flow-averaged pore diameter deduced from reported values of porosity, thickness, and water permeability.

report the porosities, 0.72–0.84, an average thickness, 138 μm, and the water bubble points of the various membranes. From their data, around membranes of cellulose esters, we construct Figure 11.3 to show the correlation between the ratings and the flow-averaged pore diameters deduced via Equation 1.8.

All the cellulosic membranes in the Nuclepore Company's Catalog Lab 50 plot as in Figure 11.3 with one exception: their 0.10-μm-rated membrane has a flow-averaged pore diameter of 0.3 μm, compared to 0.17 μm from Millipore.

11.4.1 Ratings vs. Flow-Averaged Pore Diameter

The slope of the line in Figure 11.3 is 2.0 because of the second rule of thumb given in Section 6.3: Two filter media of equal thickness where the square of the flow-averaged pore diameter in one is half that of the other show a two-fold increase of all log R values, provided the fluid velocity is the same. For example, a 0.45-μm-rated membrane with a flow-averaged pore diameter near 0.85 μm stops *B. diminuta* with log R = 3 or 4, as mentioned in Section 11.1. Another membrane of the same thickness will stop those microbes with twice the log R value when the square of the flow-averaged diameter is half that of the first membrane, that is, when the flow-averaged diameter of the second is 0.707 of the first, or 0.51 μm. Notice that in Figure 11.3 the membrane meant to stop *B. diminuta*, and rated 0.20 (or 0.22) μm, has a flow-averaged pore diameter near 0.51 μm.

If some microbes even pass the 0.20-µm-rated membrane, one proposal may be to employ a 0.10-µm-rated membrane, or, following first rule of thumb — which says that increasing the thickness of the filter medium by a factor of two results in a two-fold increase in the log R values of all particle sizes — employ two thicknesses of the 0.20-µm-rated membrane to stop them. Yet until those microbes are cultured and identified and filtration efficiency can be established, it is suggested that a 0.15-rated membrane be tried (Meltzer et al. 1999), that is, as suggested by Figure 11.3, one with a flow-averaged pore diameter of 0.45 µm.

11.4.2 Bubble Points vs. Flow-Averaged Pore Diameter

From the water bubble-point (pressures, P) of the Millipore membranes, we deduce the diameters of the largest pores, d, on a surface using (from the caption for Figure 4.1)

$$d = \frac{4\gamma}{P} \tag{11.1}$$

employing $\gamma = 72 \times 10^{-3}$ N/m, and plot those results in Figure 11.4 vs. flow-averaged pore diameters. In such a plot, we expect to see a correlation indicated by the slope of the gray line. That is we expect, from the plots in

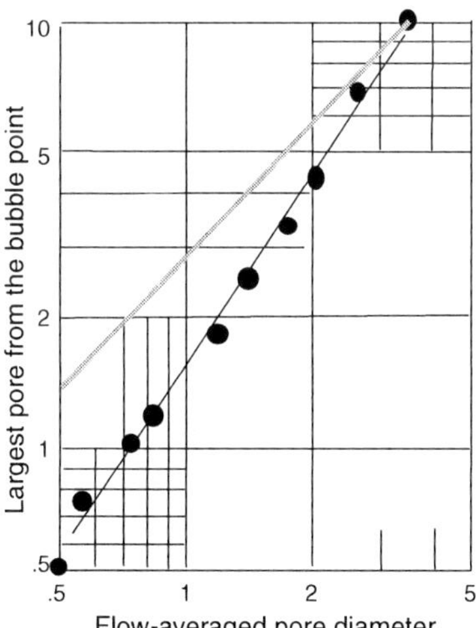

FIGURE 11.4

Another plot of Millipore data. Units of measure in micrometers, deduced from reported values of water bubble point, porosity, thickness, and water permeability. The gray line shows the theoretical correlation.

Figure 3.4, that the diameter of largest pore is at least three times that of the flow-averaged pore for all membranes. The black correlation line has a greater slope because with large-pore membranes, investigators, observing the first bubble, reach further out into the distribution than they do with small pores. That is, they see further down the wet curves in Figure 4.2, hence our plea for a standard method of measuring the bubble point.

12

Cross-Flow Filtration

12.1 What Is Cross-Flow Filtration?

In cross-flow filtration, the feed stream sweeps across the face of the filter medium rather than hitting it head on. This arrangement inhibits the accumulation of particles on the medium, thereby increasing its capacity. The simplest kind of cross-flow filtration setup is a column of liquid over a filter medium fitted with stirrer blades close to the upstream face of the medium. Particles that would otherwise settle on the medium are kept suspended in air. Such a device is generally used to test a filter medium, usually a membrane, to be installed in the kind of device schematically described in Figure 12.1. Also, Figure 12.1 shows a portion of an axial cross section of a spiral-wound tubular cartridge or module.

Alternatively, the membrane may be in the form of a bundle of hollow fibers. And, in another arrangement, the membrane may be held in a plate-and-frame kind of device. Some writers refer to this as tangential flow. Figure 12.1 is meant to show that in addition to the three streams — feed, concentrate, and permeate — we have many different pressures to consider. In correctly operated units, P_2 is, of course, greater than P_3, and P_3 is greater than P_4 and P_5, so as to make use of the full surface area of the membrane.

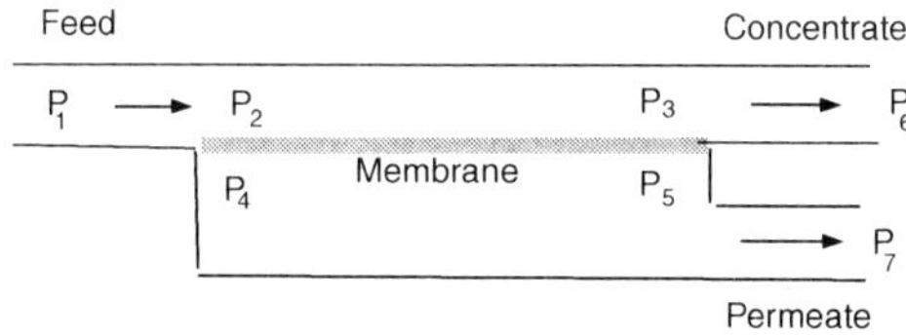

FIGURE 12.1

Schematic diagram of cross-flow filtration. Feed liquid passes over the membrane at high velocity, sweeping up particles that might accumulate on the surface and carrying them away in the concentrate stream. Meanwhile clear liquid passes through the membrane as permeate. P = pressure.

However, we only measure P_1, P_6, and P_7, which pressures may not be the same as P_2, P_3, and P_5. Given the geometry of the unit and the membrane in place, all we can do to achieve the most efficient operation is to start with a certain feed pressure, P_1, then, using valves in the two exit streams, adjust those flow rates to obtain the best results. By best, we mean not only the clarity of the permeate, however measured, relative to the feed stream but also the flow-rate ratio of permeate to feed.

12.2 Vocabulary

To discuss cross-flow filtration, we must add to — and, in some cases, change — our vocabulary. The velocity of the liquid leaving the face of the membrane, having passed through the membrane as permeate, is called flux, with the symbol J. Yet, because the word is not as specific as velocity, we continue to see and hear the term flux rate, which is akin to the land-lubber's knots per hour. We also see the redundant filtrate flux.

Filtration efficiency is referred to as rejection, or the rejection rate, or the sieving ratio. In the U.S., J is usually expressed in gal/day per square foot, the kind of units needed by the person who must calculate the area of membrane needed for the desired size of the permeate stream. Yet, not accompanying such reports are the sizes of the other streams: the feed and the concentrate. That is, conversion is not always reported.

12.3 Flow Ratios of the Three Streams

What happens to the concentrate stream? Sometimes it recirculates back to the source of the feed stream. For example, when a fermenter grows microbes, a cross-flow filter module is employed in two ways:

- During the growth of the microbes, a stream from the fermenter is fed to the cross-flow module as soluble waste products pass through the membrane as permeate, and the microbes return to the fermenter in the concentrate stream, during which time fresh nutrients are added to the fermenter.

- The final concentration of microbes in the fermenter is reached by recirculating the mixture through the cross-flow module, during which time water, with its soluble waste material, is separated as the permeate to achieved a 10-fold increase in the concentration of microbes.

Sometimes the concentrate is not recirculated to the source of the feed stream. When a module is used to reduce the salt content of water, the concentrate is discarded, while the permeate becomes the product of the operation. Before addressing the ratio of permeate flow to feed flow or to concentrate flow, we will describe the different kinds of membranes employed.

12.4 Classifications of Membranes

Membranes are classified as follows:

- When microbes or microbe-sized particles (diameters: 0.02 to 10 μm) are to be separated, the process is called microfiltration.
- When large-molecular-weight and soluble materials, such as sugars and proteins (diameters: 0.001 to 0.02 μm, or 10 to 200 Angstroms), are to be separated the process is called ultrafiltration.
- When soluble salts (diameters: 1 to 10 Angstroms) are to be separated the process is called reverse osmosis (Porter 1979).

Obviously, each of the above processes calls for a membrane with a specific flow-averaged pore size. Yet, in the case of reverse osmosis and, to some extent, in ultrafiltration, pore size is not as important as the nature of the membrane, the material of construction. Furthermore, the finer the membrane (the smaller the pores), the thinner it is produced, which enables a reasonable flux to be obtained with a reasonable driving pressure. Some very fine and thin membranes are manufactured to be used as skin on top of a coarse, support membrane. Alternatively, some membranes are formed in place within the module through the process of laying down a precoat of fine material on top of a coarser medium.

12.5 Flux Decay

Consider this set of operating conditions:

- Pressure drop across (through) the membrane
- Velocity of the feed stream across the feed stream face of the membrane
- Concentration of materials in the feed stream relative to that in the permeate

Given a certain membrane and materials to be separated from the fluid, the membrane will lose permeability with time and the flux will decay. The membrane can often be backwashed and used again, but backwashing may not restore all of the original permeability. In commercial operations, cross-flow modules are routinely backwashed and repeatedly used again but only for a finite number of cycles. The required frequency of the backwash operation depends on many factors. Indeed, if the investigator can find the proper conditions and the proper membrane, it may be minimal.

12.6 Test Procedures

Given the geometry of the module, the membrane in place, and the fluid to be filtered, only two variables remain:

- Pressure drop across (through) the membrane
- Velocity of the fluid over the feed-stream face of the membrane

One can be changed without the other by varying the feed-stream pressure and the severity with which the two exit lines are separately pinched down. Yet, pressure gauges are not located within the module, as implied by Figure 12.1. They are located in the streams feeding and emitting from the module relatively far from the membrane at points P_1, P_6, and P_7. See, for example, the diagram of a reverse-osmosis test procedure in ASTM D4516. Thus, since we really do not know the drop in pressure in the lines carrying those streams, statements about the pressure drop through the membrane and the pressure drop across the face of the membrane along the feed-stream channel are guesses. Indeed, this author has yet to see a writer assure his or her readers that in the diagram in Figure 12.1 pressures at P_2 through P_5 do indeed descend in the order they are identified.

What investigators actually measure are the differences in pressures among the three different streams. Indeed, as stated in Section 12.1, all we can do is try to find the pressure of each stream, measured close to the module, that yields the best results. Cross-membrane flow along the feed channel is referred to as shear rate, γ(1/sec). It is calculated from velocity, u, in one of two ways:

- For hollow fibers, of diameter, d, $\gamma = 8u/d$
- For rectangular slits, of height, h, $\gamma = 6u/h$

We see plots on log/log paper of flux vs. shear rate (they rise together). Yet the authors fail to state whether the plots are made with a constant pressure drop through the membrane or not.

12.7 The Boundary Layer: More on Flux Decay

As stated at the beginning of this chapter, the high velocity of the feed stream over the membrane inhibits the accumulation of solids. Nonetheless, a boundary layer forms. Ideally, we look for a layer that is thin, remains constant, and does not build up over time. Furthermore, we look for only a layer; that is, the pores in the membrane not to plug.

The composition of the layer obviously depends on the composition of the fluid. Whether or not the pores in the membrane become plugged depends on the pore sizes relative to the sizes of the solids in the feed stream and on the filtration efficiency or rejection rate. Sometimes the boundary layer is a simple, permeable cake. Other times it is so dense that the velocity (flux) of water (or solution) through it is controlled by the liquid diffusion rate. That is, no amount of extra pressure on the membrane will increase the velocity As with a dead end filter cartridge, a cross-flow module may be used in a batch operation, in which case life or capacity is not as important as it is in continuous use.

12.8 Examples of Cross-Flow Filtration

12.8.1 Reverse Osmosis

In reverse osmosis, the pressure drop through the membrane is obviously important, since it is only this pressure drop that provides the salt-rejection rate to overcome back, osmotic pressure. That is to say, in converting sea water to drinking water, high pressures are required. Yet relatively low pressures are required to convert brackish water to drinking water. Indeed, in some communities where the sodium level is high, home reverse-osmosis units employ water-line pressure to do the job but at the expense of low conversions.

For example, a home unit built to operate with, say, a 40-psi feed stream may produce 5 gallons per day of drinking water while discharging 30 gallons per day to the sewer. The conversion is 5/30 = 0.17 (17%) (ASTM D4194 and ASTM D4516).

12.8.2 Harvesting Microbes

As Norquist (1987) describes, a veterinary vaccine is produced by growing *Streptococcus pyogenes* in a 286-liter soup. After the organisms are grown to the maximum population, the mixture must be concentrated by a factor of

13 to be in the proper dosage form. To increase this concentration, a hollow-fiber module is used, containing 1 square foot of membrane surface (0.093 m^2) with a pore-size rating of 0.2 µm. Using a positive-displacement, lobe-type pump, the mixture is fed to the module at a pressure of 15 psi (1.0 bar) with outlet lines unrestricted (zero gauge pressure). The initial permeate flow of 3.5 liters/min drops to 1.9 liters/min, after which it essentially remains constant for the next 3.5 hours with a slight decay. Meanwhile the concentrate stream, returning to the fermenter, flows at an average rate of 1.0 liters/min. After 4.5 hours, with the permeate volume reaching 264 liters, the original microbe concentration in the fermenter is increased by a factor of $286/(286 - 264) = 13$.

12.8.3 Plasmapheresis

In plasmapheresis, blood under an initial driving pressure of nearly 1 mm Hg is fed to a 0.5-square-meter hollow fiber module (pore-size rating is not reported but which is designed for this procedure) at the rate of 100 liters/minute. The resulting flow of plasma as the permeate was 5 ml/min, with the remaining 95 ml/min of concentrate returning to the patient.

Over a period of four hours, the feed pressure was increased, stepwise, to 35 mm Hg, so as to maintain the feed rate at 100 ml/min. Such stepwise action increased the flow of plasma up to 35 ml/min (Werynaski et al. 1981; Malchesky et al. 1989).

12.8.4 More Examples

Johnson (1986) discusses a host of applications including wine, beer, fruit juices, suspensions of metal hydroxides, and oil and water mixtures.

12.8.5 Cross-Flow Electrofiltration

In one arrangement, a module consisting of a single hollow tube with porous walls functions as an electrode through which clarified water or oil passes. The other electrode is the wall of the module. As a direct current potential is applied across the electrodes, particles in the feed stream flowing past the porous tube are repelled. As a result, the face of the porous tube does not experience the buildup of a boundary layer. Solids suspended in either water or oil can be so treated, although oil requires more applied voltage than water. But when oil contains too many water droplets, the electrodes tend to short out. The applied polarity across the electrodes depends on the zeta potential of the suspended solids (Verdegan et al. 1985; Verdegan 1986).

12.9 Detailed Theory

Hameed and Al-Mousilly (2002), in a very theoretical analysis of fluid flow and particle size, lay out a series of about 14 steps to take in designing a cross-flow operation. They consider a short section of Figure 12.1. That is, they deal with chosen axial and suction velocities and not with changes in those velocities along the surface of the filter medium. They provide a list of 16 previous papers on the subject by a variety of authors.

13

Capacity of a Filter Medium in Constant-Pressure Filtration

13.1 Empirical Background

Capacity, in dead-end filtration, as opposed to cross-flow filtration, which we discussed in Chapter 12, refers to the volume of a specific stream or, more specifically, the amount of solids fed to a unit of area of a filter medium before the medium suffers a significant loss in permeability. Many investigators studying constant-pressure filtration make linear/linear plots of flow rate vs. time or of cumulative volume filtered vs. time. In doing so, they miss seeing what kind of empirical filtration law applies and what kind of mathematical expression describes the situation. If they had made such plots on log/log paper, where the shape of the curve is not dependent on the units of volume and time employed, they could have readily seen which law applied.

Figure 13.1 illustrates the four different shapes of curves seen when plotting cumulative volume filtered vs. time on log/log paper. Figure 13.2 illustrates the curves showing fluid-flow rate dV/dt or Q vs. time. Curve A, cake filtration, is what we hope to see. In that case, accumulated solids do not plug the pores of the filter medium; the only increasing resistance to flow is due to a growing cake of permeable solids. Figure 13.3 illustrates linear/linear plots seen around cake filtration. Curve A is parabolic. Line F, showing increased resistance with volume filtered, has twice the slope of Line E.

In Figure 13.1 or Figure 13.2, Curve D, where solids quickly plug the pores of the medium, is what we do not want to see. If we see Curve D, we can sometimes add a filter aid to the feed stream and reach Curve A or even Curves C and B. Perhaps, in a batch operation, we can live with Curves C and B or even Curve D if the area of the filter medium is consistent with the volume of fluid to be filtered.

The constant pressure test, or constant vacuum on the filtrate when it is not volatile, is the test most often performed on the laboratory bench. Aside from being simple to set up, this type of test provides the basic information from which one may predict the results of the two other kinds of tests

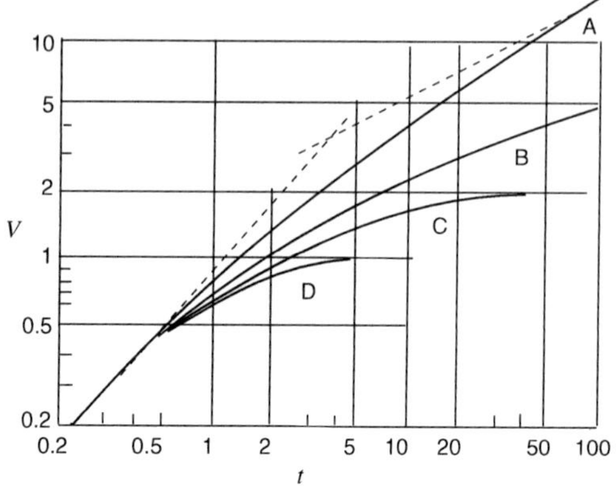

Curve	$V =$
A. Cake Filtration	$(4t + 4)^{0.5} - 2$
B. Intermediate Blocking	$\ln(1 + t)$
C. Standard Blocking	$t/(t/2 + 1)$
D. Complete Blocking	$1 - e^{-t}$

FIGURE 13.1

In constant-pressure filtration, a plot of volume filtered, V, vs. time, t, both in arbitrary units on log/log paper, generally yields a curve that follows one of four laws.

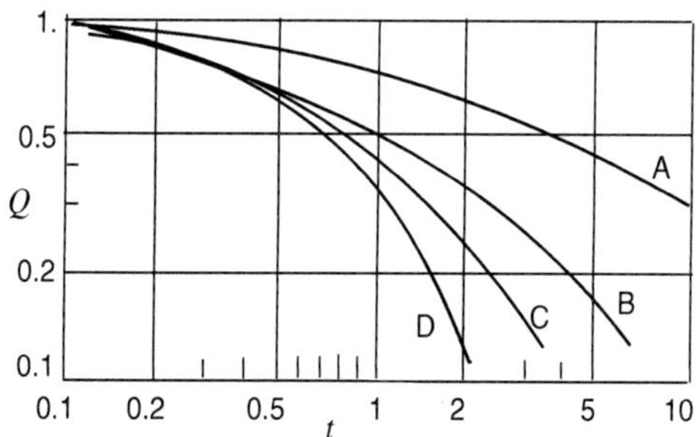

Curve	$Q =$
A. Cake Filtration	$(1 + t)^{-0.5}$
B. Intermediate Blocking	$1/(1 + 1)$
C. Standard Blocking	$(t/2 + 1)^{-2}$
D. Complete Blocking	e^{-t}

FIGURE 13.2

In constant-pressure filtration, a plot of flow-flow rate, Q, vs. time, t, in arbitrary units, illustrating four different laws.

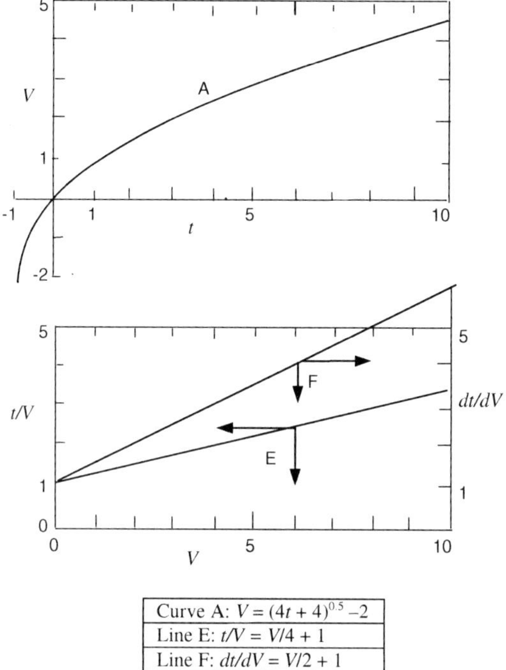

| Curve A: $V = (4t + 4)^{0.5} - 2$ |
| Line E: $t/V = V/4 + 1$ |
| Line F: $dt/dV = V/2 + 1$ |

FIGURE 13.3
Linear/linear plots of three expressions around cake filtration.

addressed in Chapter 14 and Chapter 15: (1) constant flow rate with increasing resistance and (2) varying flow and pressure, as when a centrifugal pump is employed.

The empirical, mathematical statements shown in the captions to Figure 13.1 and Figure 13.2 are normalized from more complete expressions, presented below, to show that at the start of filtration, V is a direct function of t; that is, the slopes are 1.0 and the rate constants, addressed below, are unity.

Once the filter medium begins to collect particles and offers increased resistance to flow, the flow rate, $dV/dt = Q$, usually falls according to one of the four different expressions or laws. The law with the fastest drop in permeability obviously describes Curve D. Once the filter medium begins to plug or blind it, does so quickly. Or plugging might follow Curve C or B and proceed more slowly. In either case, we obtain the measure of capacity by looking at the volume of fluid filtered when the curve takes a decided turn toward a flow rate of, say, $^1/_{10}$ the starting rate, or we just run out of time. It is a judgment call.

When the object of filtration is to recover solids or when a filter aid like diatomaceous earth has been added to the feed stream, the experimental curve may resemble Curve A. In that case the measure of capacity may be different. Capacity may be limited by the thickness of the cake of collected solids that can collect in the housing in which the medium is held in a scaled-up operation.

When the filter is a membrane, we may want to prefilter the stream with a relatively thick fibrous medium. Indeed, where a fibrous medium shows a B-, C-, or D-type of curve for a required filtration efficiency, a more open but thicker medium will show the same curve and the same filtration efficiency, yet the total volume of filtrate will be greater for a given operating time. On the other hand, it may not matter if our curve resembles Curve D, so long as the medium has the capacity for a single batch operation, after which the medium is discarded or backwashed and reused.

When a membrane is used as the final sterilizing filter, the membrane may not show a significant drop in permeability for the batch filtered, simply because the liquid is already clear of suspended solids, having been prefiltered. In any event, it is important to determine the capacity of this final filter for the liquid it will treat so that we can choose the best area of the membrane for the volume of the batch to be filtered.

13.2 Details of the Equations in Figure 13.1 and Figure 13.2

The mathematics of these equations comes from the work of Hermans and Bredée (1936), and, more completely, from Grace (1956). While the plot of data according to Figure 13.1 and Figure 13.2 provides a firsthand look at which filtration "law" was followed, other plots provide more detailed data, from which to deduce rate constants.

13.2.1 The Cake Filtration Law

The parabolic expression of Curve A in Figure 13.1 can be restated as

$$\frac{t}{V} = \frac{K_A}{2} V + \left(\frac{dt}{dV} \right)_0 \tag{13.1}$$

illustrated in Figure 13.3, as Line E. The rate constant, K_A, is the slope. On that same plot, Line F, with twice the slope, provides a measure of the increase in resistance, $1/Q$ (i.e., dt/dV), with increased V.

$$K_A V = \frac{dt}{dV} - \left(\frac{dt}{dV}\right)_0 \tag{13.2}$$

13.2.2 Intermediate Blocking

The expression for Curve B in Figure 13.1 is more fully expressed as

$$K_B V = \ln(1 + K_B Q_0 t) \tag{13.3}$$

The rate constant, K_B, is deduced from the slope in the linear/linear plot of $1/Q$ vs. t

$$K_B t = 1/Q - 1/Q_0 \tag{13.4}$$

13.2.3 Standard Blocking

To reach the rate constant Kc for Curve C, plot t/V vs. t

$$\frac{t}{V} = \frac{K_C}{2} t + \frac{1}{Q_0} \tag{13.5}$$

where the slope is $K_C/2$ and the intercept is $1/Q_0.$ Or

$$\frac{Q}{Q_0} = \left(1 - \frac{K_C V}{2}\right)^2 \tag{13.6}$$

13.2.4 Complete Blocking

The rate constant K_D, for Curve D, appears in

$$K_D V = Q_0 - Q \text{ or} \tag{13.7}$$

$$V = Q_0\left(1 - e^{-K_D t}\right) \text{ or} \tag{13.8}$$

$$Q = Q_0 e^{-K_D t} \tag{13.9}$$

13.3 Examples in Membrane Filtration

13.3.1 Expected Drop in Flow Rate or Rise in Resistance

Before discussing some experimental results, consider what we expect to see when membranes are tested and qualified to stop test microbe *Pseudomonas diminuta*. According to the photographs of Leahy and Sullivan (1978), a single, rod-shaped *Pseudomonas diminuta*, grown under specified conditions, is about 1 µm long with a diameter of about 0.4 µm. Thus, a shadow or silhouette covers an area of 0.4 µm². In testing or rating a filter membrane, 10^7 of these microbes are fed to 1 square centimeter of membrane surface, that area corresponding to 10^8 µm². Suppose these microbes lie down on the surface and do not lie on top of one another. The fraction of membrane surface covered would be $(0.4 \times 10^7)/10^8 = 0.04$. Of course, if only the pores are covered and the pores occupy 75% of the area (porosity, ε, is 0.75), the microbes will gather on the pores and 5% of the pores will be blocked. The resistance to flow will increase by a factor of $1/(1 - .05) = 1.053$. On the other hand, if the tests involve 10 times as many microbes, the resistance of the membrane will rise by a factor of $1/(1 - .5) = 2.0$.

In the case of the track-etched membrane with a porosity of only 0.1, 40% of the pore area will be covered by feeding 10^7 *Pseudomonas diminuta* per square centimeter. The resistance will rise by a factor of $1/(1 - .4) = 1.67$. However, as we will see in the next section, the resistance of each of various membranes rises much more than predicted by the above reasoning. Apparently, the broth of test microbes contains materials other than microbes to clog the pores. In any event, the examples illustrate how to address capacity in constant-pressure filtration.

13.3.2 Work of Tanny et al.

In a series of constant-pressure tests, Tanny et al. (1979) evaluated two separate cellulose-triacetate membranes for the separation of *Pseudomonas diminuta* from a broth of these freshly grown microbes. The two membranes differed only in permeability and, hence, differed only in flow-averaged pore diameters (Equation 1.8). One was rated 0.45 µm; the other, 0.20 µm. Tanny et al. fed a 2-liter broth containing about 10^8 microbes to a 47-mm-diameter filter holder, exposing them to 10.5 cm² of membrane surface or about 10^7 per square centimeter. They did this under four different driving pressures: 5, 15, 30, and 45 psi.

Figure 13.4 shows our log/log plots of volume vs. time for a driving pressure of 30 psi. The 0.20-µm-rated membrane shows a straight line with a slope of 0.5, indicating cake filtration. The curve corresponding to the 0.45-mm-rated membrane can be superimposed over Curve B in Figure 13.1, following the Standard Blocking Law. With the 0.20-µm-rated membrane, they found, as shown in Figure 13.5, that linear/linear plots of t/V vs. V essentially describe straight lines, indicating cake filtration, as in Line E in Figure 13.3. Because the filtrate was sterile in all tests at the different driving pressures, they reasoned that all microbes were captured on the surface of the membrane.

With the 0.45-μm-rated membrane, they found test microbes in the filtrate. They also found that linear/linear plots of t/V vs. t (not V), as shown in Figure 13.5, describe straight lines, not following the Standard Blocking Law. Pore blocking apparently occurred within the depths of the pores because some microbes passed through the membrane. The authors speak of adsorptive retention.

Now consider an aspect of the Cake Filtration Law not seen in the math plot of Line E in Figure 13.3. Tiller (1990a) shows that, in actual practice, Line E is not a neat straight line. When we plot the data of Tanny et al. (1979), for their 0.20-μm-rated membrane under a driving pressure of 30 psi, we obtain Curve E of Figure 13.6. To analyze that plot, draw the best straight

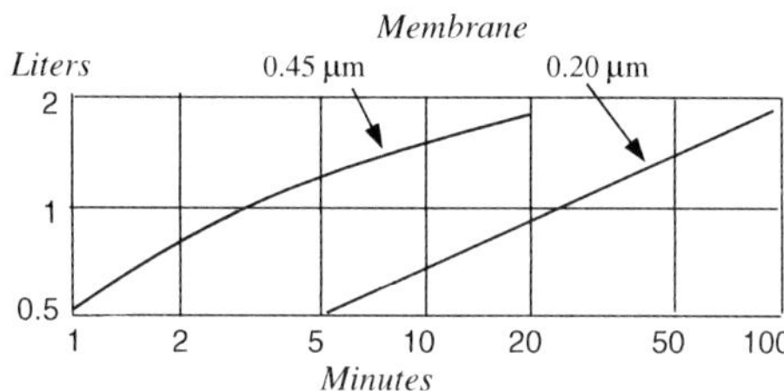

FIGURE 13.4
Plots of data from Tanny et al. (1979) on the same kind of graph paper as Figure 13.1 for driving pressures of 30 psi (207 kPa).

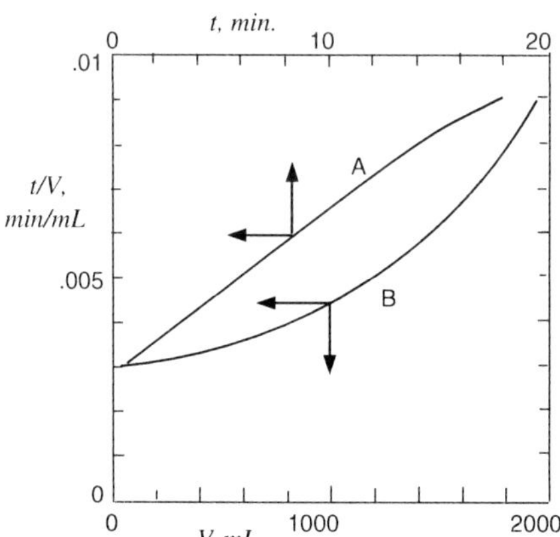

FIGURE 13.5
Plots of data from Tanny et al. (1979), for driving pressure of 30 psi (207 kPa) against a 0.45-μm-rated membrane. The straight Line A indicates the Standard Blocking Law. The Curve B indicates that cake filtration did not occur.

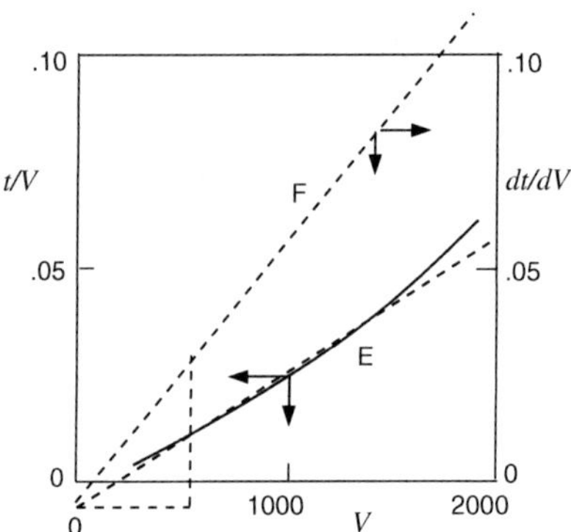

FIGURE 13.6

Plot of data from Tanny et al. (1979). Use of a 0.20-μm-rated membrane, when feeding a broth of *P. diminuta* at a driving pressure of 30 psi; *t* in minutes, *V* in milliliters. The broken Line E is drawn with the best slope. From the origin of that line, Line F is drawn with twice the slope, to indicate the increased resistance to flow.

line with a phantom origin. From that origin, draw Line F with twice the slope and thus reach a plot of increased resistance, *dt/dV*, with increased volume filtered. After 2000 ml of broth had been fed, the resistance to flow rose by a factor near 10, not the factor of 1.05 discussed in Section 13.3.1.

13.3.3 Work of Wrasidlo and Mysels

Wrasidlo and Mysels (1984) demonstrated the performance of a new type of polysulfone membrane. While an ordinary membrane of this composition is less permeable than membranes of other compositions, a polysulfone membrane with a graded porosity is much more permeable than the others. In this graded membrane, the pore size on one face is 100 times that on the other face, rated as 0.2 μm. Furthermore, the graded membrane is not only more permeable than the others, it also has a greater capacity for collecting test microbes, with the more open side receiving the feed stream. Wrasidlo and Mysels (1984) (in their Figure 9) present linear/linear plots of volume filtered, *V*, vs. time, *t*, to demonstrate this great difference. Unfortunately, for our present interest, the curve for the graded polysulfone is so crowded to the left of their plot that we cannot read the data. Yet we can read the data for the other membranes and will now examine their curves as we did those above. In these tests the investigators fed a broth of *Pseudomonas diminuta* to 25-mm-diameter membranes (area 3.5 cm²) under a driving pressure of 10 psi.

We single out two membranes, one labeled cellulosic, the other, polycarbonate (probably a track-etched membrane). Replotting their data on linear/linear coordinates, showing *t/V* vs. *t*, we obtain straight lines, following the Standard Blocking Law. The flow rate of the cellulosic membrane, after it had been fed 90 ml, dropped from 1.67 ml/sec to about 0.018 ml/sec, so that the resistance rose by a factor of 90. The flow rate of the polycarbonate membrane, after it had been fed 65 ml, dropped from 0.36 ml/sec to 0.0036 ml/sec, so that the resistance rose by a factor of 10.

13.3.4 Work of Hu et al.

Hu et al. (1993), not working with test microbes, compared a 0.2-μm-rated nylon membrane with a membrane of polyethersulfone and another of poly-vinylidene difluoride, filtering a 5% solution of bovine serum albumin. They fed this solution to 47-mm discs (about 10 cm²) at three different driving pressures and show linear/linear plots of volume filtered vs. time.

Redrawing their plots on log/log paper, we see that the curves can be superimposed over Curve C of Figure 13.1, indicating the Standard Blocking Law. The polyethersulfone membrane had twice the permeability of the other two. All other factors being equal, that membrane should have twice the capacity of the other two. In fact, it showed 2.3 to 3.0 times the capacity of the other membranes. But that capacity was only 60–85 ml per 10 cm². The point of the investigation was to show that the sulfone membrane is useful for filtering protein solutions.

13.3.5 The Silt Density Index

The silt density index (ASTM D4189) identifies a test that indirectly measures the clarity of water about to be fed to a reverse osmosis unit. It does so by determining how fast the water clogs a 47-mm diameter cellulosic 0.45-μm-rated membrane under a driving pressure of 30 psi. The test may be useful in determining the clarity of a liquid about to be fed to a 0.20-μm-rated sterilizing filter. It is easier to explain the calculations with an example than to state a formula. The test requires measuring the time to collect 500 ml from the start and then, after 5 minutes, the time to collect a second 500 ml.

Suppose the first 500 ml collects in 0.25 minute and after 5 minutes the second 500 ml collects in 0.72 minute. In this case, calculate the index as

$$\text{Silt density index} = \frac{1 - \dfrac{0.25}{0.72}}{5} \times 100 = 13.0$$

The clearer the water, the lower the index.

13.3.6 Work of Badmington et al.

Badmington et al. (1995) addressed the capacities of various membranes and sub-μm-rated prefilters during the filtration of some different liquids. Their paper describes a test procedure on a 47-mm-diameter disk of the filter medium; from the results one can determine the larger area required for the commercial volume of a liquid to be filtered.

The test procedure assumes that the filtration law one observes in action will be the Standard Blocking Law named by Hermans and Bredée (1936) and by Grace (1956) but which Badmington et al. (1995) call Gradual Blocking, even while citing the investigators who gave it its original name. The essence of the test procedure is as follows. Feed a fluid of interest to a 47-mm disk of the medium to be tested at the driving pressure of interest. Gather data regarding volume filtered, V, vs. time, t. As the test proceeds, plot t/V vs. t as in Figure 13.5 while looking for the straight line. As soon as a definite straight line appears, stop the test and determine the slope, $K_C/2$ in Equation 13.5.

Badmington et al. (1995) employed Equation 13.6 in the following steps

$$\left(\frac{Q}{Q_0}\right)^{0.5} = 1 - \frac{K_C}{2} V$$

When Q/Q_0 approaches zero, $1 = (K_C/2)V\mathrm{max}$ or $2/K_C = V\mathrm{max}$ where $V\mathrm{max}$ is the theoretical maximum volume that will filter, given enough time.

The authors seem to put great store in this $V\mathrm{max}$ test, yet mention that, in commercial practice, a filtration run is no longer sustained after Q/Q_0 falls to 0.2, or perhaps to 0.1. It would seem that instead of looking for $V\mathrm{max}$, the investigators should look for the V value — call it "$V\mathrm{practical}$" — that corresponds to, say, $Q/Q_0 = 0.15$. That is, if the specific filtration test does follow the Standard Blocking Law, then $V\mathrm{practical} = 1.225/K_C$.

13.4 Commercial Aspects of the Cake Filtration Law

In those industrial processes where solids are recovered from a slurry by filtration or where filter aids are employed, the mathematics around Curve A in Figure 13.1 have been used to calculate the resistance of the collected cake of solids. In this case we reason that the filter medium does not lose permeability. Or if it loses a little, it stabilizes with the growing cake of collected solids. We now look at how the Cake Filtration Law has been employed in these cases.

From Equation 13.2

$$\frac{dt}{dV} = K_A V + \left(\frac{dt}{dV}\right)_0$$

remembering from Figure 13.2 and Figure 13.6 how to deduce dt/dv vs. V, we obtain (Tiller et al. 1977)

$$\frac{dt}{dV} = \frac{1}{u} = \frac{\eta}{P}\left(Vc\alpha_{av} + R_m\right) \tag{13.10}$$

In the matter of units of measure, we have tried to satisfy both readers who work with English units and those who work with metric and SI units. So in Equation 13.10

t	=	time
V	=	volume of filtrate per area of filter medium, length^3/length^2
u	=	fluid-approach velocity, length/time (falls with increased V)
η	=	viscosity of the filtrate, force x time/length^2
P	=	the driving pressure, force/length^2 (held constant)
$Vc\alpha_{av}$	=	average resistance of the filter cake, 1/length (the word average reminds us that the cake immediately next to the filter medium is more resistant than the soupy cake upstream)
c	=	concentration of solids in the feed stream, mass/length^3
α_{av}	=	average specific resistance of the filter cake, length/mass, a constant for the solids under study at the pressure employed, as discussed in the last section of this chapter
R_M	=	resistance of the filter medium, 1/length, indicated by the initial resistance to flow or when a clear liquid is fed the medium

Knowing the values for all the terms in Equation 13.10 except α_{av}, solve for that constant. But understand that the constant is only specific for that pressure and the solids at hand. When the liquid-soaked solids are compressible, α_{av} will be higher at higher pressures. Indeed, to fully characterize the solids, measure α_{av} at different pressures. That is, perform constant-pressure tests at other pressures. Once having made those tests, make a plot, on log/log paper, of α_{av} vs. P. That plot (as in Figure 14.2) defines a line with a slope called the compressibility factor that tells us what to expect in constant-flow filtration as the driving pressure rises to maintain the constant flow rate.

The above cake analysis has three limitations:

- Where the concentration of solids in the feed stream is considerable so that the volume of filtrate is measurably smaller than the volume of the feed stream, V in Equation 13.10 must represent the volume of the feed stream (rather the filtrate).

- Where the solids are dense or large and settle easily, the results, which become too complicated to quantify, depend on the position of the medium, that is, whether the feed stream falls down onto a horizontal medium, flows horizontally to a vertical medium or flows up to a horizontal medium.

- Over time, fine particles in the cake sometimes migrate toward the filter medium. Thus, while we expect to see differences in the packing density of the cake from layer to layer, the migration of fine particles adds a difference in the particle-size distribution from layer to layer. This migration confounds the assumed constant meaning of α_{av} at the pressure studied.

14

Capacity of a Filter Medium in Constant-Flow Filtration

14.1 How to Test Capacity

In constant-flow filtration, capacity is usually tested on a laboratory-scale test stand with a positive-displacement pump, a flow meter, and pressure-measuring taps on the two faces of the filter medium, but the test can be performed in a pilot- or larger-scale operation. We look for increased driving pressure with elapsed time.

Driving pressure, P, is the pressure drop across the filter medium itself. If the pressure-measuring taps are located so that the measurements include pressure drop across the housing as well, one must separately measure the drop across the empty housing for the flow rate studied, then subtract that value from the drop measured across the housing with the installed medium. To immediately determine which empirical filtration law describes the situation, make a plot on log/log paper of driving pressure vs. time and compare the resulting curve to the curves of reference in Figure 14.1.

14.2 Mathematical Models of Capacity

If the experimental curve can be superimposed over Curve A, then apparently particles have been collecting on the surface of the filter medium, the pores in the medium have not plugged, and the growing cake of collected solids has remained permeable. The resistance grows with the cumulative thickness of the cake. While Curve A, as defined in the caption to Figure 14.1, never reaches a slope greater than 1.0, we do see, in operations where compressible solids are collected, that the slope is somewhat greater, as discussed below.

The mathematical statements in the caption to Figure 14.1, which define these curves, are normalized from more detailed equations in Section 14.3

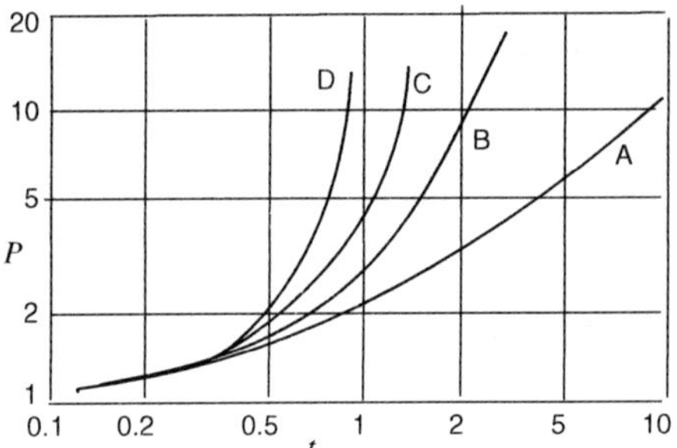

Curve	$P =$
A. Cake Filtration	$1 + t$
B. Intermediate Blocking	$\exp(t)$
C. Standard Blocking	$(1 - t)^{-2}$
D. Complete Blocking	$(1 - t)^{-1}$

FIGURE 14.1

Empirical math model plots of pressure, *P*, vs. time, *t*, in constant-flow filtration.

to show that at the start of filtration, the initial pressures and the different rate constants are unity. The fastest rise in pressure creates a plot resembling Curve D. Once the filter medium begins to plug or blind, it does so very fast. Or the filter medium may plug up somewhat more gradually, following Curve C or B. In either case, we measure capacity by looking at the volume of liquid filtered after reaching some limit of high driving pressure. It is a judgment call that depends on the initial driving pressure, which is a function of the flow rate and of the permeability of the filter medium.

Where Johnston and Schmitz (1974) and Johnston (1975) compared the performances of various tubular filters to separate black iron oxide, or silica, from water, they suggest that plots of $\log(P/P_0)$ vs. *t* on log/log paper define straight lines. The rises in pressure with time can be described by

$$\log(\log P/P_0) = \log a + b \log t$$

where *b* is the slope. Said in another way,

$$P/P_0 = \exp(at^b)$$

They found values of *b* in the range of 0.7–2.0 (compared to 1.0 for Curve B of Figure 14.1). Williams (1992), who measured the capacity of roving-wound cartridges, presents *P* vs. *t* data that when plotted on log/log paper shows curves that can be superimposed over Curve D in Figure 14.1. When the experimental curve resembles Curve A, the measure of capacity can take on a different view, as seen in those industrial processes where substantial amounts of solids are collected and which may include a filter aid. Capacity may be limited to the thickness of the cake of collected solids, defined by whatever housing holds the filter medium.

Faced with a B-, C-, or D-type curve, we may want to try to change the conditions to produce a curve that approaches Curve A. Try a finer filter medium. If the solids are not the item to be recovered, try adding a filter aid to the feed stream or precoat the aid on the filter medium or both. Try different types of filter aids and different doses to decide which to employ and at what concentration. The higher the concentration of filter aids, the more Curve A moves to the right; increased pressure is delayed. Of course, there comes a concentration when the curve no longer moves to the right as a direct function of the increased concentration of filter aid. On the other hand, we may not care if our curve resembles Curve D, so long as the medium has the capacity for a single batch operation, after which we will discard the medium or try to backwash it and use it again.

14.3 Closer Looks at the Math Models of Figure 14.1

The curves of Figure 14.1 are taken from the mathematical expressions in Grace (1956) derived from the constant-pressure expressions of Hermans and Bredée (1936). In Figure 14.1 the rate constants have been normalized; that is, rate constants and initial flow rates are unity.

To calculate rate constants, make different linear/linear plots, looking for a straight line; the slope of the line corresponds to the rate constant. In the equations to follow, P_0 = initial driving pressure, V = volume filtered, Q = volumetric flow rate, t = time, $V = Qt$, and $QV = Q^2t$.

14.3.1 The Cake Filtration Law

Plot P/P_0 vs. QV and measure the slope, K_A, in

$$P/P_0 = 1 + K_A QV \qquad (14.1)$$

14.3.2 Intermediate Blocking

Plot $\ln(P/P_0)$ vs. V and measure the slope, K_B, in

$$\ln(P/P_0) = K_B V \qquad (14.2)$$

14.3.3 Standard Blocking

Plot $(P_0/P)^{0.5}$ vs. V and measure the slope, $K_C/2$, in

$$(P_0/P)^{0.5} = 1 - (K_C/2)V \tag{14.3}$$

14.3.4 Complete Blocking

Plot P_0/P vs. V and measure the slope, K_D/Q, in

$$P_0/P = 1 - (K_D/Q)V \tag{14.4}$$

14.4 Commercial Interests in the Cake Filtration Law

Section 13.4, addressing constant-pressure filtration, explains how, once we see cake filtration, we are able to deduce the average specific resistance of the collected cake of solids. That section also mentions that when the solids are compressible, this resistance, α_{av}, is a function of the driving pressure. And, to learn if the solids are compressible, and, if so, by how much, we must perform different tests at different constant pressures.

From those test results, we make a plot on log/log paper of specific resistance, α_{av}, versus pressure, P, as illustrated in Figure 14.2 (Tiller et al. 1977). The data of such a plot are of interest in the present constant-flow test, since the driving pressure must be increased to maintain the constant flow rate.

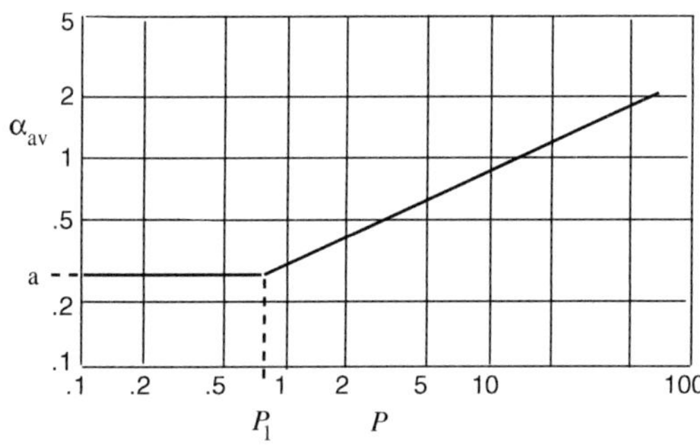

FIGURE 14.2
When solids are retained on a filter medium, following the Cake Filtration Law, repeated constant-pressure studies (separate tests at different pressures) yield data that plot like this. That is, when the solids are compressible, the average specific resistance, α_{av}, in Equation 14.5, increases with pressure, P. The slope of the line is called the compressibility factor, n in Equation 14.8. At pressures below P_1 the basic, point resistance, **a**, does not fall with decreased pressure. (Tiller et al. 1977). Measurements here are in arbitrary units.

We now derive an equation for constant-flow cake filtration, which considers how the specific resistance of the cake increases with increasing driving pressure. That is, in the absence of having done the series of constant-pressure tests to construct a plot like Figure 14.2, we can learn the compressibility from a constant-flow test by making the plot of experimental data as in Figure 14.1. On seeing a straight line develop, indicating cake filtration, we can learn the compressibility factor from the slope of that line. The greater the slope, the greater the resistance.

The basic equation in cake filtration is (Tiller et al. 1977)

$$\frac{dV}{dt} = u = \frac{P}{\eta\left(Vc\alpha_{av} + R_M\right)} \tag{14.5}$$

the terms of which are defined in Section 13.4.

When enough solids have been fed so that the pressure drop across the cake is, say, five times that across the filter medium (Curve A in Figure 14.1), neglect the resistance of the filter medium, R_M, so that Equation 14.5 becomes

$$u = \frac{P}{\eta V c\alpha_{av}} \tag{14.6}$$

Since $V = ut$, rewrite Equation 13.6 to obtain

$$P = \eta c\alpha_{av} u^2 t \tag{14.7}$$

From the results of separate constant-pressure tests, we see, from the example in Figure 14.2, that the basic or point resistance of the solids, **a**, is related to the average specific resistance, α_{av}, at a pressure P, above P_1, as follows.

$$\alpha_{av} = \mathbf{a}P^n \tag{14.8}$$

Tiller et al. (1977) explain that on integrating from P_1 to P we obtain

$$\alpha_{av} = \mathbf{a}(1 - n)(P - P_1)^n \tag{14.9}$$

Substituting Equation 14.9 into Equation 14.7 provides our working equation

$$(P - P_1)^{1-n} = \eta cu^2\alpha_{av}(1 - n)t \tag{14.10}$$

Equation 14.10 is employed as follows. On plotting experimental data as P vs. t, on log/log paper (like Curve A in Figure 14.1), measure the slope of the line where it becomes straight. Assuming P_1 is small, compared to P, neglect it (just as we assumed the pressure drop across the medium is small enough to neglect). From Equation 14.10, the slope of the line equals $1/(1 - n)$. Thus, n, the compressibility factor, equals $1 - 1/$slope. Since we know the values of all the terms in Equation 14.10, except, α_{av}, solve for α_{av} as a function of pressure.

If the slope of the P vs. t plot is 1.0 (as is Curve A in Figure 14.1), n is zero, and the cake has not compressed with increased pressure. If the slope is 3.0, then $n = 0.7$. But when n is that high, we must include P_1 in Equation 14.10 (Tiller et al. 1977) if we know it. But, of course, if we know it, by means of a Figure 14.2-type of plot, derived from different constant-pressure tests, we can predict P as a function of t.

14.5 An Example of Cake Filtration with the Use of a Filter Aid

Walton (1978, 1981), in a laboratory-scale operation, studied the use of a diatomite filter aid in clarifying beer. First laying down a precoat on the filter medium, he added this filter aid to the feed stream, calling that addition body feed. In different experiments, he used different concentrations of body feed. In Figure 1 of his 1981 paper he shows linear/linear plots of pressure vs. time. Figure 14.3 shows those data as log/log plots (as best as this writer could read Walton's linear/linear plots), from which we see the following:

- Without body feed (with only the precoat), Curve 1 is a straight line with a slope of 1.09.
- With body feed, Curve 2 has a little bend, with an average slope of 1.3. Curve 3, with a little more bend, has an average slope of 1.18.
- With more body feed, Curve 4, comes the realization that only so much body feed is useful.

The mass concentration of solids in the beer was determined by passing a sample of beer through a 0.45-μm-rated, cellulose-ester membrane and weighing the solids, to calculate the gravimetric level. Those solids, of yeast cells and organic debris, were present at a mass concentration of 140 parts per million. The precoat level consisted of 0.15 pound of diatomite per square foot of filter area. In analyzing Walton's data, use Equation 14.10, which states that a log/log plot of P vs. t should be a straight line, from which deduce the compressibility factor, n, and the average cake resistance, α_{av}.

What follows is an abbreviated way of analyzing data. Since Walton does not report the viscosity of the filtrate, η, we look at the term $\eta\alpha_{av}$ in Equation 14.10 as one unit, calling it α, and will analyze Curves 2 and 3.

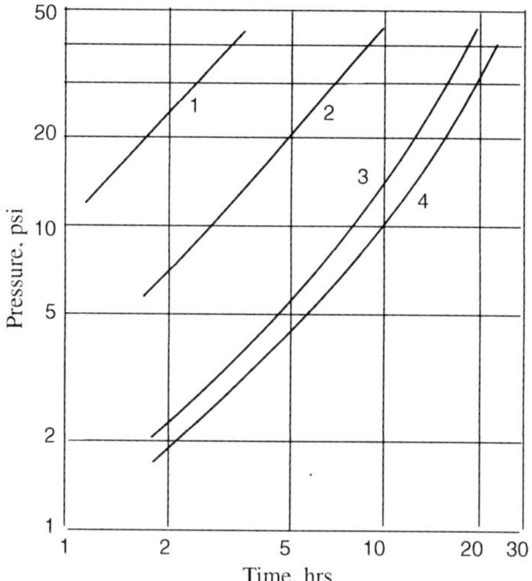

FIGURE 14.3

Data of Walton (1978, 1981), here plotted on log/log paper, employing diatomite filter aid to clarify beer. Curve 1: No body feed, only a precoat of filter aid on the filter medium. With the addition of body feed, the ratios of filter aid to the mass of solids in the beer were: Curve 2: 2/1; Curve 3: 3/1; Curve 4: 4/1.

14.5.1 Curve 2

With an average slope of 1.1, so that $n = 1 - 1/1.1 = 0.0909$, solve for α when $P = 6.0$ psi, and $t = 2$ hrs, using Equation 14.10.

$$P^{1-n} = (1 - n)\alpha t$$

$$\alpha = \frac{P^{1-n}}{(1-n)t} = \frac{6.0^{0.902}}{0.909 \times 2} = 2.80 \text{ units of resistance}$$

After $t = 10$ hrs, when P has risen to 45 psi, the resistance of the cake, α, has risen to 3.43 units.

14.5.2 Curve 3

With more body feed, the cake has less resistance, and the pressure rise is delayed. With an average slope of 1.21, so that $n = 1 - 1/1.21 = 0.174$, while $n - 1 = 0.826$, calculate α at the two ends of the curve.

When $P = 2.0$ psi and $t = 2$ hrs, $\alpha = 1.073$

When $P = 40$ psi and $t = 20$ hrs, $\alpha = 1.27$

14.6 General Comments

In constant-rate, cake filtration, there exists an optimum rate for obtaining the most volume of filtrate and collecting the most mass of solids during a cycle (Purchas 1977). The time required for constant-rate filtration is twice that of constant-pressure filtration to reach the same volume of filtrate and the same pressure (Purchas 1977; Tiller et al. 1977).

15

Capacity of a Filter Medium in Variable-Pressure and Variable-Flow Filtration

15.1 Centrifugal Pumps

When a stream feeding a filter medium is moved by a centrifugal pump, the system rides the pump curve. As the filter medium loses permeability, more back pressure on the pump results in a decreased flow rate. When a sand bed is used to clarify water, the driving force is the column of water over the bed. Flow out the bottom of the bed is controlled by a valve so that, as the bed looses permeability, the valve opens more, trying to maintain a constant flow. But eventually as the bed plugs and the valve opens all the way, the flow rate falls to the point where the bed must be backwashed before operations can be resumed.

Just as we constructed the mathematical model plots of Figure 13.1 for constant-pressure filtration and the plots of Figure 14.1 for constant-flow filtration, we can construct such plots for variable-pressure and variable-flow filtration. Just as Figure 13.1 shows four different models of volume filtered, V, vs. time, t, for constant driving pressure, and Figure 14.1 shows pressure, P, vs. t, for constant flow rate, Figure 15.1 shows the ratio of V/P vs. t when both pressure and flow rate change over time.

Tiller (1990a, 1990b) provides an example of cake filtration with a centrifugal pump. If we make a time plot of his changing ratio of volume filtered to pressure on log/log paper, such a curve can be superimposed over Curve A in Figure 15.1 as illustrated in Figure 15.2. In those situations where laboratory filtration tests are done at many different constant pressures (Chapter 13), Tiller et al. (1977) explain how to predict the results of employing a centrifugal pump, knowing the pressure/flow relationship of the pump.

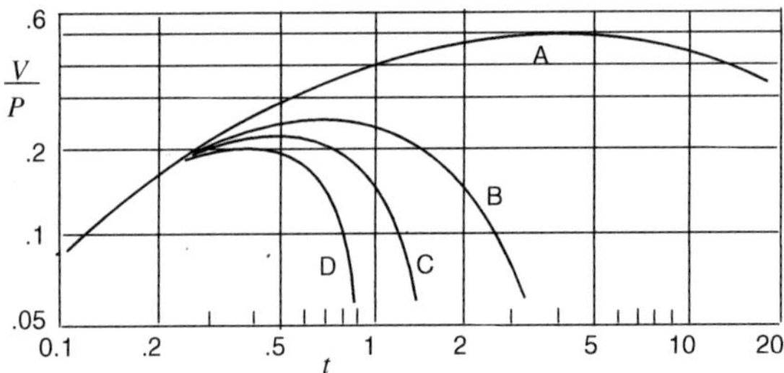

FIGURE 15.1
The types of results seen when a centrifugal pump feeds liquid to a filter medium. Combinations of the two separate groups of mathematical models in Figure 13.1 (volume, V vs. time, t, in constant-pressure filtration) and Figure 14.1 (pressure, P vs. t, in constant-flow filtration). A = cake filtration, B = intermediate filtration, C = standard blocking, D = complete blocking.

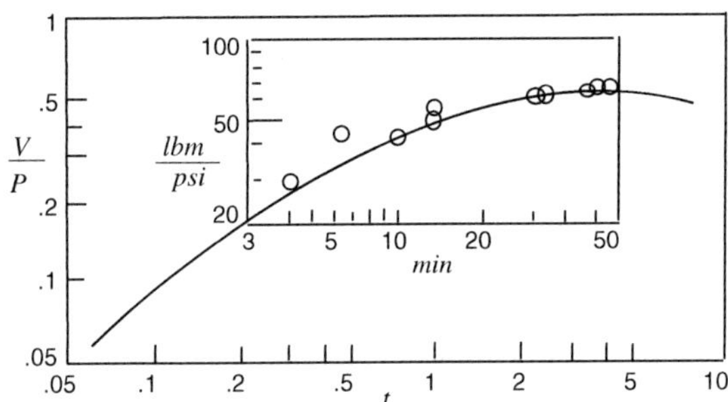

FIGURE 15.2
The inner frame shows a plot of data from Tiller (1990b) from the filtration of cottonseed oil. The outer frame shows Curve A of Figure 15.1.

15.2 An AIChE Test Procedure

Another test procedure for centrifugal pump situations is provided by AIChE (1967), which explains how to determine the resistance of the filter cake with increased driving pressure when both the flow rate and driving pressure change over time. In one example, a 500-sq-foot plate-and-frame filter is fed a water slurry containing 0.003 mass fraction of talc. Thus, in the terms below, the talc concentration, c, is 0.187 lbm/ft^3. The tabulated operating data of this example are plotted here as the curves of Figure 15.3. The viscosity, η, of the 43°F filtrate is 1.47 cP, equal to $3.07 \cdot 10^5$ lbf·sec/ft^2. From the data of Figure 15.3, we construct Table 15.1, and thus calculate the average specific resistance of the cake, α_{av}, with increased pressure, in units of 10^{11} ft/lbm.

Table 15.1 shows that α_{av} increases with increased driving pressure. In a log/log plot of α_{av} vs. P (not shown here), the slope is not significantly

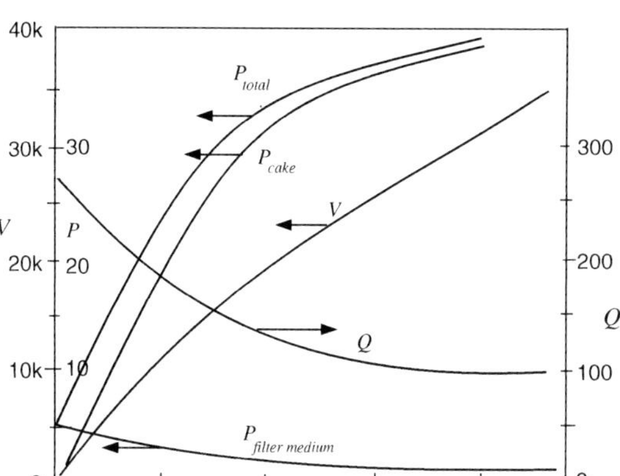

FIGURE 15.3

Plot of data tabulated in AIChE (1967). In this example a 500-sq-foot plate-and-frame filter is fed a slurry of talc via a centrifugal pump at a changing flow rate, Q gal/min. Assuming cake filtration, the pressure drop across the medium, P_{medium} psi, decreases with decreased flow rate. Hence, from the increased total driving pressure, P_{total}, the increasing pressure across the cake P_{cake} is calculated as the volume of filtrate, V gallons, increases.

TABLE 15.1

Analyses of Data from Figure 15.3

Time, min.	25	50	100	150
gal/min	234	180	130	95
u, 10^{-4} ft/sec	10.4	8.0	5.77	4.04
Pc, psi on cake	11	19.5	32	35
P, lbf/ft²	1,584	2,808	4,608	5,040
gallons	5,800	9,000	17,000	24,000
V, ft³/ft²	1.55	2.40	4.54	6.43
$\alpha_{av} = P/Vc\eta u$	1.70	2.55	3.06	3.38

different from 0.51, the compressibility factor of talc reported by Tiller et al. (1977). Yet the authors of these AIChE data do not address the obvious questions concerning the end of the run. When the flow rate leveled off instead of dropping, did some of the cake fall off the filter medium? Did a portion of the filter medium give way? Chase (1993) addresses the size of a centrifugal pump to be used.

15.3 A Draw-Down or Recirculation Scheme of Filtration

We discuss the subject of draw-down or recirculation filtration in this chapter because it may be performed with a centrifugal pump. Liquid is drawn from a container and passed through a filter, and the filtrate is continuously returned to the container. During the run, both the feed stream and the filtrate are periodically examined by whatever analytical method we use to find out about the concentration of undesirable particles. For example, we may look at turbidity or the concentration of d-diameter particles or the mass concentration of all particles (the gravimetric level). Or we may only examine the feed stream to the filter, which represents the bulk of the liquid in the container when the contents of the container are well stirred.

While gathering the analytical data during the run, we begin making a plot where the vertical axis, a log scale, shows the concentration of whatever we measured in the feed stream. Knowing the volume of liquid in the container and the volumetric flow rate through the filter, we construct the horizontal axis on a linear scale to show time, but marking that time scale as the numbers of turnovers. For example, if we have 100 gallons of liquid in the container and pump 10 gal/min through the filter, we have one turnover in 10 minutes, two in 20 minutes. If the liquid in the container is well stirred and filtration efficiency, however we measure it, remains constant, the plot will show a straight line with a negative slope. The slope describes the rate at which the liquid in the container becomes clearer over time. The more negative the slope, the greater the filtration efficiency.

Joseph (1994) shows a plot of such theoretical conditions where the vertical scale is linear, in which case we see falling, concave curves.

While Hong (1985) shows log scales for the vertical axis in his plots of experimental data, and falling straight lines occur, the lines then curve out. Hong measured the clarity of the liquid feeding the filter by the National Fluid Power Association (NFPA) method. That is, instead of looking at the concentration of d-diameter particles, he looked at the concentration of the numbers of d-diameter-and-larger particles. Hong actually followed the NFPA multipass test procedure but without the continued addition of test dust to the feed tank. He calls his test Beta prime.

15.4 Supercompactable Filter Cakes

Tiller et al. (2002) studied the filtration of sludges from the effluents of sewage disposal plants. In lab tests, they increased the driving pressures in steps while monitoring the flow-rate and found that above a certain driving pressure solids were compacted to the degree that flow stopped. Those critical pressures were in the range of 2 to 9 psi, yet the solids content of the cakes was no more than twice that of the feed stream. They concluded that further deliquoring would have to be done by means of a belt press or centrifugation. Some processes simply dry the sludge into pellets.

References

AIChE. 1967. *Equipment Testing Procedure Batch Pressure Filters*. American Institute of Chemical Engineers, New York.

Alderete, J. 1991. A practical approach to filtration ratings and effective filter selection. Memo DOR1606, Cuno, Inc., Meriden, CT.

ASTM D3862. 1980. *Retention Characteristics of 0.2-μm Membrane Filters Used on Routine Filtration Procedures for the Evaluation of Microbiological Water Quality*. ASTM, West Conshohocken, PA.

ASTM D3863. 1987. *Retention Characteristics of 0.40- to 0.45-μm Membrane Filters Used on Routine Filtration Procedures for the Evaluation of Microbiological Water Quality*. ASTM, West Conshohocken, PA.

ASTM D4189. 1982. *Silt Density Index of Water*. ASTM, West Conshohocken, PA.

ASTM D4194. 1985. *Operating Characteristics for Reverse Osmosis Devices*. ASTM, West Conshohocken, PA.

ASTM D4195. 1988. *Water Analysis for Reverse Osmosis Application*. ASTM, West Conshohocken, PA.

ASTM D4516. 1985. *Practice for Standardizing Reverse Osmosis Performance Data*. ASTM, West Conshohocken, PA.

ASTM E128. 1989. *Maximum Pore Diameter/Permeability of Rigid Filters*. ASTM, West Conshohocken, PA.

ASTM F316. 1986. *Pore Size Characteristics of Membrane Filters by Bubble Point and Mean Flow Pore Test*. ASTM, West Conshohocken, PA.

ASTM F660. 1983. *Particle Size Comparisons in Use of Alternative Particle Counters*. ASTM, West Conshohocken, PA.

ASTM F778. 1988. *Standard Methods for Gas Flow Resistance Testing of Filtration Media*. ASTM, West Conshohocken, PA.

ASTM F795. 1988. *Performance Testing of a Filter Medium Using a Single-Pass, Constant-Rate Liquid Test*. ASTM, West Conshohocken, PA.

ASTM F796. 1988. *Performance Testing of a Filter Medium Using a Single-Pass, Constant-Pressure, Liquid Test*. ASTM, West Conshohocken, PA.

ASTM F797. 1988. *Performance Testing of a Filter Medium Using a Multi-Pass, Constant-Rate Liquid Test*. ASTM, West Conshohocken, PA.

ASTM F838. 1983. *Bacterial Retention of Membrane Filters Utilized for Liquid Filtration*. ASTM, West Conshohocken, PA.

ASTM F902. 1984. *Average Circular-Capillary Equivalent Pore Diameter in Filter Media*. ASTM, West Conshohocken, PA.

ASTM F1215. 1989. *Initial Particle Size Efficiency of Flatsheet Medium in an Airflow, Using Latex Spheres*. ASTM, West Conshohocken, PA.

ASTM. 1986. *STP [Special Technical Publication] 975: Fluid Filtration. Vol. I, Gas; Vol. II, Liquid*. ASTM, West Conshohocken, PA.

Badenhop, C.T. 1983. *The Determination of the Pore Distribution and the Consideration of Methods Leading to the Prediction of Retention Characteristics of Membrane Filters.* Dr. Ing Dissertation, University of Dortmund, Germany. Available from UMI (University Microfilms), Ann Arbor and London.

Bader, H. 1970. Hyperbolic distribution of particle sizes. *J. Geophysical Research* 75:2822–2830.

Badmington, F. 1995 with R. Wilkins, M. Payne, and E.S. Honig. Vmax testing for practical microfiltration train scale-up in biopharmaceutical processing. *Pharm. Tech.* Sept:64–76.

Bear, J. 1972. *Dynamics of Fluids in Porous Media.* Elsevier, New York.

Bliesner, W.C. 1964. A study of the porous structures of fibrous sheets using permeability techniques. *Tappi J.* 47(7):392–400.

Bocquet, P.C. 1951 (translator). Two monographs on Electrokinetics. Helmholtz: Studies on electric boundary layers. Schmoluchowski: Electric endosmosis and streaming potential. *Engineering Research Bulletin 33.* Engineering Research Institute, University of Michigan, Ann Arbor.

Bower, J.P. 1986. Correlation of biologic retention latex particle retention and physical tests on 0.1 micron pore rated membrane filters. In *ASTM STP 975,* Vol II. ASTM, West Conshohocken, PA. 51–58.

Brittain, H.G. 2002. Particle-size distribution. Part III Determination by analytical sieving. *Pharm. Tech.* Dec:56–64.

Campbell, J.S. 1981 with M. Iwanaga. Beta rating variation with different test contaminants. *The BFPR Basic Fluid Power Research Program Journal* 14:87–93.

Carman, P.C. 1937. Fluid flow through granular beds. *Transactions Institute of Chemical Engineers London* 15:150–166.

Carman, P.C. 1956. *Flow of Gases through Porous Media.* Butterworths, London.

Chase, G.G. 1993. Accounting for pipe loss when comparing centrifugal pumps for your filtration. *Fluid/Particle Separation J.* 6:84–89.

Cheap, D.W. 1982. Leaf tests can establish optimum rotary-vacuum-filter operation. *Chem. Eng.* June 14:141–148.

Cole, F. 1966. *Particle Count Rationalization.* Bendix Filter Division, Madison Heights, MI.

Conner, W.C. 1984 with A.M. Lane and A.J. Hoffman. Measurements of the morphology of high surface area solids: histeresis in mercury porosimetry. *J. Colliod and Interfacial Science* 100:186–193.

Corte, H.L. and E.H. Lloyd. 1966. Fluid flow through paper and sheet structure. In F. Bolan (Ed.), *Consolidation of the Paper Web.* British Paper and Board Makers Assoc., London. 981–1009.

Coyne, K.W. 1986 with W.C. Conner and K. Rucinski. Filter morphology and performance: porosity and microscopy of oil filter media compared with filtration. *Chem. Engineer* 32:53–62.

D'Andrea, T. 2003. Filter performance: practical aspects of filter ratings. *Filtration News* Mar/Apr:14, 16, 18, 21.

Davies, C.N. 1973. *Air Filtration.* Academic Press, New York.

Dickenson, C. 1992. *Filters and Filtration Handbook.* Elsevier Science Publishing Co., Oxford.

Dodson, C.T.J. 1996 with W.W. Sampson. The effect of paper formation and grammage on its pore-size distribution, *J. Pulp and Paper Science* 35(3):287–292.

Dodson, C.T.J. 1997 with W.W. Sampson. Modeling a class of stochastic porous media, *Appl. Math. Letters* 10(2):87–89.

Dullien, F.A.L. 1979. *Porous Media Fluid Transport and Pore Structure*. Academic Press, New York. 159–161.

Eleftherakis, J.G. 1998 with I. Khalil. Multipass beta filtration testing for the 21st Century, *Fluid/Particle Separation J.* 11(3):351–356.

Elford, W.J. 1933. The principles of ultrafiltration as applied to biological studies. *Proc. Royal Soc.* 112B:384–406.

Ergun, S. 1952. Fluid flow through packing columns. *Chem. Eng. Progress* 48:89–94.

Fitch, R.C. 1970. *Supplemental Report 70-1 of the Basic Fluid Power Research Program Annual Report*. Oklahoma State University, Stillwater.

Francis, T. 1992. *Arizona Test Dust Update*, Powder Technology Inc., Burnsville, MN.

Grace, H.P. 1956. Structure and performance of filter media, *AIChE J.* 2:307–336.

Graham, K. 2002 with M. Ouyang, T. Raether, T. Grafe, B. McDonald, and P. Knauf. Polymeric nanofibers in air filtration applications, *15th Annual Technical Conference and Expo of the American Filtration and Separation Society,* Galveston, TX, April. 9–12.

Grant, D.C. 1988. *Sieving Capture of Particles by Microporous Membrane Filtration Media*. Master's thesis, University of Minnesota, Minneapolis.

Grant, D. 1990 with J.G. Zahka. Sieving capture of particles by microporous membrane filters from clean liquids. *Swiss Contamination Control* 3:160–164.

Green, L. 1951 with P. Duwez. Fluid flow through porous metals. *J. Applied Mechanics* 18:39–45.

Hameed, M.S. 2002 with D.S. Al-Mousilly. Design of a crossflow filtration system. *Filtration & Separation*. June:45–47.

Haring, R.E. 1970 with R.A. Greenkorn. A statistical model of a porous medium with nonuniform pores. *AIChE J.* 16:477–483.

Hermans, P.H. 1936 with H.L. Bredée. Principles of the mathematical treatment of constant-pressure filtration. *J. Soc. Chem. Industry* 55:T1–4.

Hernandez, A. 1996 with J.L. Calvo, P. Pradanos, and F. Tejerina. Pore size distributions in microporous membranes: a critical analysis of the bubble point extended method. *J. Membrane Science* 112:1–12.

Hofmann, F. 1984. Testing of microfiltratration membranes. *J. Parenteral Science and Technology* 38:148–159.

Hong, I.T. 1985. The beta prime — a new advanced filtration theory. *Filtration & Separation* July/Aug: 235–238.

Hu, H.J. 1993 with J. Camilleri and W. Tamashire. A new membrane for biopharmaceutical filtration. *Pharm. Tech.* Oct:30, 34, 36, 38, 40, 42, 44.

Jaisinghani, R. 1982 with B. Verdegan. Electrokinetics in hydraulic oil filtration — the role of anti-static additives. *World Filtration Congress III, Vol. II*, Filtration Society (UK). 618–626.

Jaroszczyk, T. 1985 with T. Ptak. Experimental study of aerosol separation using a minicyclone. *10th Annual Powder & Bulk Solids Conference*, Rosemont, IL.

Jaroszczyk, T. 1987a. Vortex dust feeder for industrial research, Filtech Conference, Utrecht.

Jaroszczyk, T. 1987b. Experimental study of nonwoven filter performance using second order orthogonal design. *Particulate Science and Technology* 5:271–287.

Jaroszczyk, T. 1987c with R.H. Hoops and G. Kreikebaum. Measurements of air efficiency using a continuous aerosol monitoring system. *SAE Paper 872268*. Dearborn, MI.

Jaroszczyk, T. 1991 with J. Wake. Critical aerosol velocity in nonwoven filtration. *TAPPI Nonwoven Conference*, Atlanta.

Johnson, B.R. 1990 with SK. Herweyer; E.M. Johnson, and J.K. Agarwal. A new automated filter tester for low eficiency, HEPA grade and above filter media and cartridges. *Bulletin ITI 012*, TSI, Inc., St. Paul, MN.

Johnson, E.M. 1990 with B.R. Johnson, and S.K. Herweyer. A new CNC based automated filter tester for fast penetration testing of HEPA and ULPA filters and filter media. *Bulletin ITI 016*, TSI, Inc., St. Paul, MN.

Johnson, J.N. 1986. Crossflow microfiltration using polypropylene hollow fibers. In *ASTM STP 975*. ASTM, West Conshohocken, PA. 15–26.

Johnston, P.R. 1974 with J. Schmitz. A new and recommended way to view the test performance of cartridge filters. *Filtration & Separation* Nov/Dec: 581–585.

Johnston, P.R. 1975. Submicron filtration. *Chem. Eng. Progress (CEP)* 17:70–73.

Johnston, P.R. 1976. Number and weight distributions of particles in streams around filters. *Filtration & Separation* Mar/Apr:134–136.

Johnston, P.R. 1978. The particle-size distribution in AC fine test dust. *J. Testing & Eval.* 6:103–107.

Johnston, P.R. 1979 with T. Meltzer. Comments on the organism-challenge levels in sterilizing-filter efficiency testing. *Pharm. Tech.* 3:66–70, 110.

Johnston, P.R. 1980 with T. Meltzer. Suggested integrity testing of membrane filters at a robust flow of air. *Pharm. Tech.* 4(11):49–51.

Johnston, P.R. 1982a. Determining the average pore diameter in tubular filter cartriges (candles) from fluid permeability measurements. *World Filtration Congress III, Vol. I*. Filtration Society, UK. 591–595.

Johnston, P.R. 1982b with R. Swanson. A correlation between the results of different instruments used to determine the particle-size distribution in AC fine test dust. *Powder Technology* 32:119–124.

Johnston, P.R. 1983. The most probable pore size distribution in filter media. I. Evidence of such a distribution from results of extended bubble-point measurements. *J. Testing & Eval*, 11 (2):117–121.

Johnston, P.R. 1985. Fluid filter media: measuring the average pore size and the pore-size distribution, and correlation with results of filtration tests. *J. Testing & Eval.* 13(4):308–315.

Johnston, P.R. 1989. The viscous permeability of a mat of randomly arrayed fibers as function of fiber diameter and packing density. *Fluid/Particle Separation J.* 2:15–16.

Johnston, P.R. 1992. *Fluid Sterilization by Filtration*, 1st ed. Interpharm Press, Engelwood, CO.

Johnston, P.R. 1995. *A Survey of Test Methods in Fluid Filtration*, Gulf Pub. Co., Houston.

Johnston, P.R. 1997. *Fluid Sterilization by Filtration*, 2nd ed, Interpharm Press, Engelwood, CO (now CRC Press).

Johnston, P.R. 1998a. Comments on fluid-intrusion measurements for determining the pore-size distribution in filter media. *Filtration & Separation* 35(5):455–459.

Johnston, P.R. 1998b. *Fundamentals of Fluid Filtration: A Technical Primer*, 2nd ed. Tall Oaks Pub. Co., Littleton, CO.

Johnston, P.R. 1998c. Revisiting the most probable pore-size distribution. The gamma distribution. *Filtration & Separation* 35(3):287–292.

Johnston, P.R. 1999a. Clearly determine the best filter medium. *Chem. Eng. Progress (CEP)* June:73–79.

Johnston, P.R. 1999b. *Statistical Methods Demystified: A Practical Primer for Engineers and Scientists*. LLH Technology Publishing.

Johnston, P.R. 2000. Understand particle-size distributions when testing filter media. *Chem. Eng. Progress* Mar:47–50.

Jornitz, M. 2001 with T.H. Meltzer. *Sterile Filtration, a Practical Approach*. Marcel Dekker, New York.

Joseph, J.J. 1994. Pilot testing liquid clarification equipment by progressive dilution. *Filtration News* Mar/Apr:44–45.

Leahy, T.J. 1978 with M.J. Sullivan. Validation of bacterial retention capabilities of membrane filters. *Pharm. Tech.* 2:65–75.

Liu, B.Y.H. 1986 with K.L. Rubow. Air filtration by fibrous media. In *ASTM STP 975*. Vol. I. ASTM, West Conshohocken, PA. 1–74.

Macdonald, I.F. 1979 with M.S. El-Sayed, K. Mow, and F.A.L. Dullen. Flow through porous media — the Ergun Equation revisited. *Industrial Eng. Fundamentals* 18:199–208.

Malchesky, P.S. 1989 with T. Horiuchi, J.J. Lewandowski, and Y. Nos. Membrane plasma separation and the on-line treatment of plasma by membranes. *J. Membrane Science* 44:55–88.

McBroom, K. 1993. Conversation with Peter Johnston.

McKinnon, B.T.K. 1993 with K. Avis. Membrane filtration of pharmaceutical solutions. *Amer. Hosp. Pharm.* 50:1921–1936.

Meltzer, T.H. 1987. *Filtration in the Pharmaceutical Industry*. Marcel Dekker, New York.

Meltzer, T.H. 1999 with M. Jornitz and P. Johnston. Relative efficiencies of double filters or tighter filters for small-organism removals. *Pharm. Tech.* Sept 98:100, 102, 104.

Meyer, B.A. 1985 with D.W. Smith. Flow through porous media: comparison of consolidated and unconsolidated materials. *I&EC Fundamentals* 24:360–368.

Miller, B. 1986 with I. Tyomkin. An extended range liquid extrusion method for determining pore size distributions. *Textile Research J.* 56:35–40.

Millipore Corp. 1971. Catalogue MC/1. Bedford, MA.

Monson, D.R. 1986. Key parameter used in modeling pressure loss of fibrous filters. In *ASTM STP 975*, Vol. I. ASTM, West Conshohocken, PA. 27–45.

NFPA. 1990. ANSI/NFPA T3.10.8.8 RI. (ISO 16889, 1999). *Hydraulic Fluid Power Filters: Multi-Pass Method for Evaluating Filtration Performance*. National Fluid Power Association, Milwaukee.

Norquist, R. 1987. Solving liquid/solids separation problems with hollow fiber, cross-flow microfiltration. In *Pharmaceutical Filtrations*. Society of Manufacturing Engineers, Dearborn, MI.

Nuclepore Corp. 1980. Catalog Lab50, Pleasanton, CA.

Omokawa, S. 1991 with P.S. Malchesky, J.B. Goldcamo; S.R. Savon, and Y. Nos. Immunomodulating effects of serum-material interactions. *J. Biomedical Materials Research* 25:621–636.

Oulman, C.S. and R.E. Baumaner, 1970. Streaming potential in diatomite filtration of water. *J. Am Water Works Assoc.* 56:915–30; *Filtration & Separation* Nov/Dec:682.

Pall, D.B. 1978 with E.A. Kirnbauer. Bacteria removal prediction in membrane filters. Presented at the 52nd Colloid and Surface Science Symposium, University of Tennessee, Knoxville. Copy available from Pall Corp.

Piekaar, H.W. 1967 with L.A. Clarenburg. Aerosol filters — pore size distribution in fibrous filters. *Chem. Eng. Science* 22:1399–1408.

Pierce, M. (no date) with R. Guimond and N. Lifshutz. A general correlation of DOP penetration with face velocity as function of particle dize using the FTS-200. *Bulletin ITI 014*, TSDI, Inc., St. Paul, MN.

Porter, M.C. 1979. Membrane filtration. In *Separation Technology for Chemical Engineers.* P.A. Schweitzer (Ed.). McGraw-Hill, New York.

Purchas, D.B. 1977. *Solid/Liquid Separation Equipment Scale-up.* Uplands Press, Croydon, England.

Remiarz, R. (no date) with B.R. Johnson, and J.K. Agarwal. Automated systems for filter efficiency measurements. *Bulletin ITI 002.* TSI, Inc., St. Paul, MN.

Reti, A.R. 1977. An assessment of test criteria in evaluating the performance and integrity of sterilizing filters. *Bull. Parenteral Drug Assoc.* 31:187–194.

Rosenstein, N.D. 1980 with A. Dybbs, and R.V. Edwards. *Non Linear Laminar Flow in a Porous Medium.* Publication FTAS/TR-80–148, Dept. of Mechanical and Aerospace Engineering, Case Western Reserve University, Cleveland.

Rubow, K.L. 1986 with B.Y.H. Liu. Characteristics of membrane filters for particle collection. In *ASTM STP 975,* Vol. I. ASTM, West Conshohocken, PA. 74–94.

Rushton, A. 1977 with P.V.R. Griffiths. Chapter 3 of *Filtration Principles and Practice, Part I.* Clyde Orr (Ed.). Marcel Dekker, New York.

SAE. 1988. J1858. *Full Flow Lubricating Oil Filters Multipass Method for Evaluating Filtration Performance.* Society of Automotive Engineers, Warrendale, PA.

Sampson, W.W. 2001. Comments on the pore-radius distribution in near-planar stochastic fibre networks. *J. Material Science,* 36:5131–5135.

Scheidegger, A. 1963. *The Physics of Flow through Porous Media.* University of Toronto Press, Toronto.

Schroeder, H.G. 1986 with J.A. Simonetti and T.H. Meltzer. Prediction of filtration efficiency from integrity test data. In *ASTM STP 975.* ASTM, West Conshohocken, PA. 27–50.

Simpson, K.L. 1989 with S.G. Iverson. A comparison of two NaCl test systems used for measuring filter efficiency. *Bulletin ITI 017,* TSI, Inc., St. Paul, MN.

Sueoka, A. 1983 with P.S. Malchesky. Particle filtration for determination of pore size characteristics of microporous membranes: Applicability to plasma separation membranes. *Separation Science and Technology* 18:571–584.

Suthar, A. 2002 with G. Chase. Performance of meltblown media with nanofibers. *Fluid/Particle Separation J.* 14 (2):58–64.

Tanny, G.B. 1979 with D.K. Strong, W.G. Presswood, and T.H. Meltzer. Adsorptive retention of *Pseudomonas diminuta* by membrane filters. *J. Parenteral Drug Assoc.* 33:40–51.

Tepper, F. 2002 with L. Kaledin, S.R. Farrah, and J. Lukasik. Nanosize fiber depth filter. *15th Annual Technical Conference and Exposition of the American Filtration and Separation Society,* Galveston, TX.

Tiller, F.M. 1977 with A. Alciatore and M. Shirato. Chapter 5 of *Filtration Principles and Practice, Part I.* C. Orr (ed.). Marcel Dekker, New York.

Tiller, F.M. 1990a. Tutorial: Interpretation of filtration data. I. *Fluid/Particle Separation J.* 3:85–94.

Tiller, F.M. 1990b. Tutorial: Interpretation of filtration data, II, Pilot plant filtration of cottonseed oil. *Fluid/Particle Separation J.* 3:157–164.

Tiller, F.M. 2002 with W. Li and S. Jeane. Characterizing the super-compactability of wastewater filter cakes. *15th Annual Technical Conference and Exposition, American Filtration and Separation Society,* Galveston, TX.

Treybal, R. 1980. *Mass-Transfer Operations.* McGraw-Hill, New York.

Trotter, A.M., 2002 with O. Rodrigues and L. Thomas. The usefulness of 0.45 μm-rated filter membranes. *Pharm. Tech.* Apr:60, 62, 64, 66, 68, 70.

Trottier, R.A. 1990 with R.C. Brown 1990. The effect of aerosol charge and filter charge on the filtration of submicrometer aerosols. *Bulletin ITI 0921*, TSI, Inc., St. Paul, MN.

VanOsdell, D. 1986 with R.P. Donovan. Electrostatic enhancement of fabric filters. In *ASTM STP 975*, Vol. I. ASTM, West Conshohocken, PA. 316–331.

Verdegan, B.M. 1985 with J. Draxler and H. Fenrick. Field dependence of particle electrophoretic mobility on non-polar liquids. *Particulate Science & Technology* 3:115–126.

Verdegan, B.M. 1986. Cross-flow electrofiltration of petroleum oils. *Separation Science & Technology* 21:603–623.

Verdegan, B.M. 1992 with K. McBroom and L. Liebman. Recent developments in oil filter test methods. *Filtration & Separation* July/Aug.

Walton, H.G. 1978. Laboratory procedure and filter for diatomite filtration tests. *Filtration & Separation* Jan./Feb.

Walton, H.G. 1981. Diatomite filtration — optimising the body feed. *Filtration & Separation*. (Photocopy).

Wallhäusser, K.H. 1979. Is the removal of microorganisms by filtration really a sterilization method? *J. Parenteral Drug Assoc.* 33:156–170.

Washburn, E.W. 1921. The dynamics of capillary flow. *Physical Reviews.* 17:273–282.

Werynaski, A. 1981 with P.S. Malchesky, A. Sucoka, Y. Asanuma, J.W. Smith, K. Kayashima, E. Herpy, H. Sato, and Y. Nos. Membrane plasma separation toward improved clinical operation. *Transactions of the American Society of Artificial Internal Organs* XXVII:539–543.

Williams, C.J. 1992. Testing the performance of spool-wound cartridge filters. *Filtration & Separation* Mar/Apr:162–168.

Willis, M.S. and I. Tosun. 1980. A rigorous cake filtration theory. *Chem. Eng. Science* 35:2427–2438.

Worthy, W. 1984, Electric separation tested in phosphate settling ponds. *Chem. & Eng. News (CEP)*, Jan 30:23.

Wrasidlo, W. 1984 with K.J. Mysels. The structure of some properties of graded highly asymmetrical porous membranes. *Parenteral Science and Technology* 38:24–31.

Yavorsky, D. 2002. The clarification of bioreactor cell cultures for biopharmaceuticals. *Pharm. Tech.* Mar:62–76.

Yukawa, H., et al. 1971. Fundamental study of electroosmotic filtration. *J. Chem. Eng. of Japan*, 4:370–376.

Zeman, L. 1982 with G. Tkacik. 1982. Pore volume distribution in ultrafiltration nembranes. *Amer. Chem. Soc. Symposium Series*, No. 269:339–350.